Veggie Delights

Title:

Veggie Delights:

A Collection of Mouthwatering Vegan Recipes.

BY

Tony Irving.

Veggie Delights

Veggie Delights

Table of Contents:

Contents

Chapter 1: Breakfast Bliss Start your day with energy and flavor. From fluffy vegan pancakes with fresh berries to savory tofu scrambles and creamy overnight oats, these breakfast recipes will make you look forward to your mornings.

Chapter 2: Appetizing Appetizers Elevate your gatherings with these appetizers that burst with flavor. Try the stuffed mushroom caps, crispy avocado bites, and zesty buffalo cauliflower wings – perfect for parties or a casual snack.

Chapter 3: Sensational Soups Warm your soul with hearty vegan soups. Whether you're in the mood for a classic tomato soup, a spicy Thai coconut curry, or a comforting lentil stew, these recipes will satisfy your cravings.

Chapter 4: Savory Salads Discover the art of salad-making with creative and satisfying vegan salads. From a colorful quinoa and roasted vegetable salad to a fresh Mediterranean-inspired bowl, these salads are anything but boring.

Chapter 5: Pasta Perfection Indulge in rich and creamy pasta dishes that are entirely plant-based. Creamy cashew Alfredo, roasted red pepper pesto, and spicy arrabbiata – these recipes will make you forget about traditional dairy-based sauces.

Chapter 6: Hearty Vegan Mains Explore the versatility of plant-based proteins with these main dishes. Enjoy a spicy chickpea curry, a comforting vegan shepherd's pie, or a flavorful vegetable stir-fry.

Chapter 7: Side Dish Delights Complement your meals with delightful vegan side dishes. These recipes will steal the spotlight, from garlic-roasted Brussels sprouts to buttery mashed sweet potatoes and herbed quinoa.

Chapter 8: Decadent Desserts Satisfy your sweet tooth without compromising on your vegan lifestyle. Dive into decadent chocolate avocado mousse, creamy coconut rice pudding, or a classic apple crisp with a vegan twist.

Chapter 9: International Flavors In this chapter, we embark on a global culinary journey to explore the rich and diverse world of international vegan dishes. From savory Moroccan tagines to spicy

Indian curries, and Italian pasta classics, these recipes bring the flavors of the world to your kitchen.

Chapter 10: Hearty Vegan Bowls Bowls are a popular trend in contemporary cuisine, and in this chapter, we take it to the next level with Hearty Vegan Bowls. Discover nourishing Buddha bowls, vibrant grain bowls, and protein-packed power bowls that are as visually appealing as they are delicious.

Veggie Delights

Dedication:
To Vegans all over the world.

Veggie Delights

Copyright
© 2023 by Tony Irving

All rights reserved. No part of this publication may be reproduced, distributed, or transmitted in any form or by any means, including photocopying, recording, or other electronic or mechanical methods, without the prior written permission of the author, except in the case of brief quotations embodied in critical reviews and certain other noncommercial uses permitted by copyright law.

Cover Design by Tony Irving

Disclaimer
The views and opinions expressed in this book are those of the author and do not necessarily reflect the official policy or position of any organization or entity mentioned within. Any resemblance to actual persons, living or dead, or actual events is purely coincidental.

Notice of Liability
The information in this book is distributed on an "As Is" basis, without warranty. While every precaution has been taken in the preparation of this work, neither the author nor the publisher shall have any liability to any person or entity with respect to any loss or damage caused or alleged to be caused directly or indirectly by the information contained in this book.

Synopsis:

"Veggie Delight" is a culinary masterpiece that invites beginners and seasoned chefs alike to enter the vibrant world of plant-based cuisine. Across ten engaging chapters, this cookbook promises a delightful exploration of diverse vegan dishes that satisfy the senses and nourish the body.

The journey begins with "Chapter 1: Breakfast Bliss" which includes a vibrant collection of delicious vegan breakfast recipes that will help you add flavor, energy, and good health to your day, while "Chapter 4: Savory Salad" adds a bit of pizzazz to the repertoire, setting the tone for the rest of the book. Each subsequent chapter opens up on a unique theme, from "Delicious Appetizers" to "Sensational Soups" and "Pasta Perfection" to demonstrate the versatility and richness of botanical ingredients.

"Chapter 6: "Hearty Vegetarian Dishes" and the climax of the book in "Chapter 10: Hearty Vegan Bowls provide nutritious options for those looking for hearty meals and a perfect ending that refreshes the palate and leaves a lasting impression. Throughout the chapters, recipes come to life with careful instructions, allowing home cooks and seasoned chefs alike to create delicious, eye-catching dishes. Each dish is not only a treat for the taste buds, but also a celebration of a sustainable and compassionate lifestyle.

In short, "Veggie Delight" pushes the conventional boundaries of vegan cuisine, proving that plant-based meals can be as satisfying, if not more, than regular meals. This engaging cookbook is filled with diverse and appealing recipes, encouraging a shift towards more compassionate, healthier, and more environmentally friendly eating. With "Veggie Delight", the future of the culinary world appears to be not only green but also extremely delicious. Wishing you happy and delicious cooking!

Tips and Tricks for Cooking and Life:

The tips and tricks in this cookbook cover both cooking and life-related scenarios. They can help to make you more skilled and efficient in your cooking, while also making you able to manage your everyday life.

Cooking Tips:

i. **Read Recipes Thoroughly:** Before you start any recipe, ensure you read it from start to finish to understand the steps and gather all the ingredients and equipment needed.

ii. **Mise en Place:** Prior to starting to cook, prepare all your needed ingredients (chopping, measuring, etc.). This will make your cooking process a smooth one.

iii. **Taste as You Go:** Taste and adjust your dishes as you cook along. Adjust seasoning as you need to get your desired flavor.

iv. **Learn Knife Skills:** Investing in time to improve your knife skills is key. It will make slicing, chopping, and other knife jobs easier and safer.

v. **Use a Timer:** Set timers to avoid overcooking or burning dishes.

vi. **Keep Your Pans Hot:** Heat up the pans before you add ingredients. This is to ensure proper cooking and to prevent sticking.

vii. **Rest Meat:** Allow cooked meat to rest before cutting to retain juices and tenderness.

viii. **Master Basic Techniques:** Invest time to Learn basic techniques like roasting, sautéing, and braising in order to have a wide range of dishes.

ix. **Stock Essentials:** Always have some basic staples like broth, onions, canned tomatoes, and garlic on hand for easy meal preparation.

Life Tips:

i. **Plan Ahead:** Stay organized by prioritizing tasks. Have to-do lists to plan your day.

ii. **Practice Mindfulness:** learn to reduce stress and improve mental well-being by incorporating mindfulness exercises into your routine.

iii. **Stay Hydrated:** Drink enough water throughout the day for better energy and overall health.

iv. **Exercise Regularly:** Embed physical activity into your daily routine. This will boost your mood, reduce stress, and improve fitness.

v. **Manage Finances:** Always have a budget. Set financial goals and track your spending to achieve it.

vi. **Embrace Learning**: Continuously seek opportunities to learn and acquire new skills or knowledge.

vii. **Simplify and Declutter:** Regularly declutter and simplify your living space to reduce stress and improve focus.

viii. **Practice Gratitude:** Happiness is free. Learn to dwell and reflect more on the positive side of your life. This will improve your happiness and mental well-being.

Benefits of Following Tips and Tricks:

i. **Efficiency:** If you follow these tips and tricks, you will save time and effort in both cooking and everyday tasks. You will achieve more in less time.

ii. **Skill Improvement:** Implementing cooking tips will make you a better, more skilled, and confident cook who creates delicious meals with ease.

iii. **Better Health:** Using tips like meal planning and fresh ingredients while cooking at home, you will develop healthier eating habits and better nutrition.

iv. **Stress Reduction:** Organization and mindfulness are life management tips that can reduce stress and improve overall well-being.

v. **Financial Well-Being:** Financial tips can help you budget, save, and invest wisely, leading to improved financial stability.

vi. **Personal Growth:** Continuously learning and applying new tips and tricks can contribute to personal growth and self-improvement.

vii. **Sustainability:** Cooking and life tips can include eco-friendly practices that contribute to a more sustainable and environmentally friendly lifestyle.

viii. **Improved Quality of Life:** Following tips and tricks can lead to a more enjoyable and fulfilling life by enhancing various aspects of daily living.

If you make these tips and tricks a part of your cooking and life, they can bring about positive changes, making your culinary and personal life journey more successful, efficient, and enjoyable.

Chapter 1:

Breakfast Bliss.

The first rays of sunlight gently caress your face as you wake up to the promise of a brand-new day. There's something magical about the morning, and it's even more enchanting when you know you're about to indulge in a sumptuous, plant-based breakfast. Chapter 1 of "Veggie Delights" is all about Breakfast Bliss – a collection of mouthwatering vegan breakfast recipes that will kick start your day with flavor, energy, and wholesome goodness.

1. Fluffy Vegan Pancakes:

The aroma of freshly cooked pancakes wafts through the kitchen as golden-brown discs sizzle on the griddle. These pancakes are light, airy, and every bit as satisfying as their non-vegan counterparts. The secret ingredient? Aquafaba, the liquid from a can of chickpeas, creates the perfect egg replacement, giving the pancakes that coveted fluffiness. Top them with a drizzle of pure maple syrup and a handful of ripe berries, and you have a breakfast worth savoring.

How to Prepare:

Ingredients:

i.   1 cup all-purpose flour

ii.   2 tablespoons sugar

iii.   2 teaspoons baking powder

iv.   1/2 teaspoon salt

v.   1 cup almond milk (or any plant-based milk of your choice)

vi.   2 tablespoons vegetable oil (or melted coconut oil)

vii.   1 teaspoon vanilla extract

viii.   Cooking spray or extra oil for greasing the pan

Instructions:

i.   In a mixing bowl, whisk together the flour, sugar, baking powder, and salt.

ii.   In a separate bowl, combine the almond milk, vegetable oil, and vanilla extract.

iii.   Pour the wet ingredients into the dry ingredients and stir until just combined. It's okay if there are a few lumps; overmixing can make the pancakes tough.

iv.   Preheat a non-stick skillet or griddle over medium heat. Lightly grease it with cooking spray or a small amount of oil.

v.   Pour 1/4 cup of the pancake batter onto the skillet for each pancake. Cook until bubbles form on the surface, and the edges start to look set, usually about 2-3 minutes.

vi.   Flip the pancakes and cook for an additional 1-2 minutes, or until they are golden brown and cooked through.

vii.   Remove the pancakes from the skillet and keep them warm while you cook the remaining batter.

viii.   Serve your fluffy vegan pancakes with your favorite toppings, such as maple syrup, fresh fruit, vegan butter, or nuts.

Benefits of Vegan Pancakes:

i.   **Plant-Based:** Vegan pancakes are entirely free of animal products, making them suitable for vegans and vegetarians. This choice aligns with a plant-based lifestyle, which can have several health and environmental benefits.

ii.   **Lower in Saturated Fat:** Traditional pancakes often contain butter and eggs, which are high in saturated fat. Vegan pancakes use healthier fats, like vegetable oil, which can help lower saturated fat intake.

iii.   **Cholesterol-Free:** Vegan pancakes don't contain cholesterol, which can contribute to better heart health.

iv.   **Rich in Fiber:** Depending on the type of flour used, vegan pancakes can be a good source of dietary fiber, aiding digestion and promoting a feeling of fullness.

v. **Allergen-Friendly:** Vegan pancakes are suitable for people with dairy or egg allergies, making them a safe and delicious option for those with dietary restrictions.

vi. **Customizable:** You can customize vegan pancakes with a variety of toppings like fresh fruit, nuts, seeds, or vegan chocolate chips, making them a versatile and nutritious breakfast option.

Keep in mind that the nutritional content of your pancakes may vary depending on the specific ingredients you use, so it's a good idea to check the labels on your chosen products to ensure they align with your dietary goals.

2. Savory Tofu Scramble:

For those who prefer a savory start to their day, the tofu scramble is a game-changer. Tofu, crumbled and seasoned with turmeric and nutritional yeast, mimics the texture and taste of scrambled eggs without the cholesterol or cruelty. Add diced bell peppers, onions, and spinach for a burst of color and flavor. Serve it on whole-grain toast or alongside some crispy hash browns for a hearty and satisfying breakfast.

Veggie Delights

How to Prepare:

Ingredients:

i. 1 block (14 oz or 400g) firm tofu, drained and crumbled

ii. 1 tablespoon olive oil or vegetable oil

iii. 1/2 small onion, finely chopped

iv. 1 bell pepper, diced

v. 2 cloves garlic, minced

vi. 1/2 cup cherry tomatoes, halved

vii. 1/2 cup spinach or kale, chopped (optional)

viii. 1/2 teaspoon turmeric powder (for color)

ix. 1/2 teaspoon cumin powder

x. 1/2 teaspoon paprika

xi. Ensure salt and black pepper are to your taste

xii. 2 tablespoons nutritional yeast (optional, for a cheesy flavor)

xiii. Fresh parsley or cilantro, for garnish (optional)

Instructions:

i. Heat the olive oil in a large skillet or frying pan over medium heat.

ii. Add the chopped onions and bell peppers. Sauté for about 3-4 minutes until they start to soften.

iii. Add the minced garlic and continue to sauté for another minute until fragrant.

iv. Add the crumbled tofu to the skillet, along with the turmeric, cumin, paprika, salt, and black pepper. Stir well to evenly coat the tofu with the spices. Cook for about 5-7 minutes, stirring occasionally, until the tofu is heated through and begins to take on a golden color.

v. Toss in the cherry tomatoes and spinach (or kale) if using. Cook for an additional 2-3 minutes until the tomatoes start to soften, and the spinach wilts.

vi. If you want a cheesy flavor, sprinkle nutritional yeast over the tofu scramble and stir to combine. Cook for another minute to let the flavors meld.

vii. Taste the scramble and adjust the seasoning if necessary.

viii. Remove the skillet from heat, garnish with fresh parsley or cilantro if desired, and serve hot.

Benefits of Savory Tofu Scramble:

i. **High Protein:** Tofu is a rich source of plant-based protein, making this scramble a satisfying and protein-packed breakfast or brunch option.

ii. **Low in Saturated Fat:** Tofu is low in saturated fat, making it a heart-healthy protein source.

iii. **No Cholesterol:** Tofu is cholesterol-free, which is beneficial for heart health.

iv. **Rich in Nutrients:** This dish is rich in essential nutrients, including vitamins, minerals, and antioxidants from the vegetables and spices used.

v. **Versatile:** You can customize your tofu scramble with various vegetables and spices to suit your taste preferences.

vi. **Dairy-Free:** This recipe is entirely dairy-free and suitable for those with lactose intolerance or a dairy-free diet.

vii. **Filling and Satisfying:** This dish's combination of protein and vegetables can help keep you feeling full and satisfied throughout the morning.

viii. **Low in Calories:** Depending on the portion size and added ingredients, tofu scrambles can be a relatively low-calorie breakfast option, making them suitable for those watching their calorie intake.

Enjoy your savory tofu scramble as a delicious and nutritious breakfast or brunch dish!

3. Creamy Overnight Oats:

Busy mornings call for convenience, and that's where overnight oats shine. Simply mix rolled oats with your favorite plant-based milk, a touch of sweetener, and a medley of fresh or dried fruits, then refrigerate overnight. By morning, you'll have a creamy, cold, and nutritious breakfast ready to devour. Experiment with toppings like sliced bananas, chopped nuts, chia seeds, or a dollop of almond butter for added texture and flavor.

How to Prepare:

Ingredients:

i. 1/2 cup rolled oats
ii. 1/2 cup plant-based milk (such as almond milk, soy milk, or oat milk)
iii. 1/4 cup Greek yogurt (or a dairy-free alternative)
iv. 1-2 tablespoons maple syrup or honey (adjust to taste)
v. 1/2 teaspoon vanilla extract
vi. A pinch of salt
vii. Add any toppings you choose (fresh berries, bananas, nuts, seeds, a drizzle of nut butter)

Instructions:

i. In a mixing bowl or a mason jar, combine the rolled oats, plant-based milk, Greek yogurt, maple syrup (or honey), vanilla extract, and a pinch of salt.

ii. Stir everything together until well combined.

iii. Seal the bowl or jar with a lid and refrigerate it overnight or for at least 4 hours to allow the oats to absorb the liquid and soften.

iv. In the morning, give the oats a good stir. If the mixture is too thick for your liking, you can add a little more milk to achieve your desired consistency.

v. Top your creamy overnight oats with your favorite toppings. Common choices include fresh berries, sliced bananas, chopped nuts, seeds (like chia seeds or flaxseeds), or a drizzle of nut butter.

Enjoy your creamy overnight oats cold, straight from the fridge. If you prefer them warm, you can microwave them for a short time to heat them.

Benefits of Creamy Overnight Oats:

i. **Convenient Breakfast:** Overnight oats are a quick and convenient breakfast option, as they can be prepared the night before and are ready to eat in the morning, saving you time.

ii. **Nutrient-rich:** Oats are a good source of dietary fiber, vitamins, and minerals. They can help keep you full and provide sustained energy throughout the morning.

iii. **Digestive Health:** The fiber in oats can support digestive health by promoting regular bowel movements and maintaining gut health.

iv. **Protein:** Greek yogurt adds a protein boost to your overnight oats, making them more satisfying and helping with muscle repair and maintenance.

v. **Dairy-Free Option:** This recipe can easily be made dairy-free by using plant-based milk and dairy-free yogurt, making it suitable for those with lactose intolerance or a vegan diet.

vi. **Customizable:** You can personalize your overnight oats with a variety of toppings, allowing you to create different flavor combinations to suit your taste preferences.

vii. **Natural Sweetener:** Maple syrup or honey provides sweetness without the need for refined sugar, making this a healthier breakfast option.

viii. **Versatile:** You can experiment with different flavors by adding ingredients like cocoa powder, spices (cinnamon, nutmeg), or extracts (almond, coconut) to create unique variations.

Creamy overnight oats are delicious and a nutritious way to start your day, providing a balanced mix of carbohydrates, protein, and healthy fats.

4. Vegan French Toast:

Imagine thick slices of bread soaked in a flavorful, eggless batter and cooked to golden perfection. That's vegan French toast for you! The batter is made using plant-based milk, a hint of vanilla, and a touch of cinnamon, creating a fragrant and delightful coating for your bread. Serve it with a dusting of powdered sugar, a drizzle of agave nectar, and a side of fresh fruit for a breakfast that feels like a decadent treat.

How to Prepare:

Ingredients:

i. 4 slices of thick bread (such as sourdough, whole wheat, or French bread)
ii. 1 cup unsweetened almond milk (or any plant-based milk of your choice)
iii. 2 tablespoons chickpea flour (also known as besan)
iv. 2 tablespoons maple syrup or agave syrup
v. 1 teaspoon vanilla extract
vi. 1/2 teaspoon ground cinnamon

vii.   A pinch of salt

viii.   Cooking oil or vegan butter for frying

ix.   Toppings of your choice (e.g., fresh fruit, maple syrup, powdered sugar, vegan whipped cream)

Instructions:

i.   In a mixing bowl, whisk together the almond milk, chickpea flour, maple syrup, vanilla extract, ground cinnamon, and a pinch of salt until well combined. This mixture serves as your vegan "egg" batter.

ii.   Heat a non-stick skillet or frying pan over medium-high heat and add a small amount of cooking oil or vegan butter to grease the pan.

iii.   Dip each slice of bread into the vegan "egg" batter, ensuring both sides are coated evenly. Allow any excess batter to drip off.

iv.   Place the coated bread slices in the hot skillet and cook until golden brown on both sides, usually about 3-4 minutes per side. You may need to adjust the heat to prevent burning.

v.   Transfer the cooked vegan French toast to a plate.

vi.   Serve your vegan French toast with your favorite toppings, such as fresh fruit, maple syrup, powdered sugar, or vegan whipped cream.

Benefits of Vegan French Toast:

i. **Cruelty-Free:** Vegan French toast is free from eggs and dairy, making it a compassionate choice for those who follow a vegan lifestyle or have dairy and egg allergies.

ii. **Lower in Saturated Fat and Cholesterol:** Unlike traditional French toast, which uses eggs and butter, vegan French toast is lower in saturated fat and contains no cholesterol, which can contribute to better heart health.

iii. **Plant-Based Nutrients:** Plant-based milk, such as almond milk, can provide essential nutrients like calcium, vitamin D, and vitamin B12 (if fortified).

iv. **Fiber:** Depending on the type of bread you choose, vegan French toast can be a source of dietary fiber, which supports digestive health.

v. **Customizable:** You can personalize your vegan French toast with a variety of toppings and spices, allowing you to create unique flavor combinations.

vi. **Natural Sweeteners:** This recipe uses natural sweeteners like maple syrup or agave syrup instead of refined sugar, which can be a healthier choice.

vii. **Versatile:** You can adapt the recipe to your dietary preferences and needs by choosing the type of plant-based milk and bread that suits you best.

Vegan French toast provides a delicious and satisfying breakfast option while offering the benefits of being cruelty-free, lower in saturated fat, and customizable to your taste. Enjoy it as a special treat or a regular morning indulgence.

5. Fruit-Filled Smoothie Bowls:

Sometimes, simplicity is the ultimate luxury. Smoothie bowls are a fantastic way to load up on vitamins and nutrients while enjoying a refreshing, customizable breakfast. Blend your favorite fruits, greens, and plant-based yogurt or milk, then top it with a delightful assortment of toppings like granola, coconut flakes, and fresh berries. It's a visually appealing and nutritious way to start your day.

How to Prepare:

Ingredients:

Smoothie Base:

i. 1 1/2 cups frozen mixed berries (strawberries, blueberries, raspberries, etc.)
ii. 1 ripe banana
iii. 1/2 cup unsweetened almond milk (or any plant-based milk of your choice)
iv. 1/2 cup Greek yogurt (or a dairy-free alternative)
v. 1 tablespoon honey or maple syrup (optional, for added sweetness)

Toppings:

i. Sliced fresh fruit (e.g., berries, kiwi, banana)
ii. Granola
iii. Chopped nuts (e.g., almonds, walnuts)
iv. Seeds (e.g., chia seeds, flax seeds)
v. Coconut flakes
vi. Additional honey or maple syrup for drizzling (optional)

Instructions:

i. Prepare the Smoothie Base:
ii. In a blender, combine the frozen mixed berries, ripe banana, almond milk, Greek yogurt, and honey or maple syrup (if using).
iii. Blend until smooth and creamy. If the mixture is too thick, add a bit more

almond milk to reach your desired consistency.

iv.   Assemble the Smoothie Bowl:

v.   Pour the smoothie base into a bowl.

vi.   Arrange your choice of sliced fresh fruit, granola, chopped nuts, seeds, and coconut flakes on top of the smoothie base.

vii.   Drizzle with additional honey or maple syrup if you prefer extra sweetness.

viii.   Serve immediately and enjoy your fruit-filled smoothie bowl!

Benefits of Fruit-Filled Smoothie Bowls:

i.   **Nutrient-Rich:** Fruit-filled smoothie bowls are packed with a variety of vitamins, minerals, and antioxidants from fruits, nuts, seeds, and other toppings. These nutrients support overall health and well-being.

ii.   **Fiber:** The combination of whole fruits and toppings like granola and seeds provides dietary fiber, which aids in digestion and helps you feel fuller for longer.

iii.   **Protein:** Greek yogurt, if used, adds a protein boost to the smoothie bowl, which is important for muscle repair and satiety.

iv.   **Hydration:** The base of the smoothie bowl is made with almond milk and fruits, contributing to hydration due to their water content.

v. **Customizable:** You can tailor your smoothie bowl to your taste and dietary preferences. Choose your favorite fruits and toppings to create endless flavor combinations.

vi. **Energy Boost:** This breakfast is a great way to start your day with a burst of energy from the natural sugars in the fruits and carbohydrates from the toppings.

vii. **Vegan Option:** To make this recipe vegan, simply replace Greek yogurt with a dairy-free yogurt alternative and use maple syrup instead of honey.

viii. **Visual Appeal:** Smoothie bowls are not only delicious but also visually appealing, making them an enjoyable and Instagram-worthy breakfast option.

Including fruit-filled smoothie bowls in your diet can be a delicious and nutritious way to boost your intake of fruits, fiber, and essential nutrients, helping you maintain a balanced and healthy lifestyle.

Conclusion:

Chapter 1 of "Veggie Delights" invites you to celebrate the beauty of breakfast with a vegan twist.

Veggie Delights

These recipes not only cater to your taste buds but also align with your ethical and health-conscious choices. Whether you're craving something sweet or savory, these Breakfast Bliss creations will make your mornings brighter and your journey into plant-based eating a joyful one. Start your day right with the magic of vegan breakfasts!

Chapter 2:

Appetizing Appetizers.

Appetizers set the stage for any meal, igniting the palate and teasing the taste buds with flavors that promise a delicious culinary journey ahead. In Chapter 2 of "Veggie Delights," we delve into the world of Appetizing Appetizers, offering you a treasure trove of plant-based creations that are perfect for gatherings, parties, or simply elevating your everyday snacking experience.

1. **Stuffed Mushroom Caps:**

Picture plump, earthy mushroom caps stuffed with a savory mixture of breadcrumbs, herbs, garlic, and vegan cheese. These stuffed mushroom caps are baked to perfection, creating a delightful combination of crispy tops and tender interiors. They make for an elegant and irresistible appetizer that will impress both vegans and omnivores alike.

How to Prepare:

Ingredients:

- 12 large button mushrooms.
- 1/2 cup breadcrumbs (plain or seasoned)
- 1/4 cup grated Parmesan cheese (or a vegan alternative).
- 2 cloves garlic, minced
- 2 tablespoons fresh parsley, chopped

Veggie Delights

- 2 tablespoons olive oil
- Salt and black pepper to taste

Optional: additional grated cheese for topping

Instructions:

i. Preheat your oven to 375°F (190°C).

ii. Remove the mushrooms stems carefully and set them aside. Then gently twist and wiggle the stems to loosen them from the caps.

iii. In a bowl, combine the breadcrumbs, grated Parmesan cheese (or vegan alternative), minced garlic, chopped parsley, olive oil, salt, and black pepper. Mix well until you have a moist, crumbly filling.

iv. Take each mushroom cap and stuff it generously with the breadcrumb mixture. Press the filling gently into the cap to ensure it sticks.

v. If desired, sprinkle additional grated cheese on top of each stuffed mushroom cap.

vi. Place the stuffed mushroom caps on a baking sheet or in a baking dish.

vii. Bake in the preheated oven for about 15-20 minutes or until the mushrooms are tender and the filling is golden brown and crispy.

viii. Remove from the oven and let them cool for a few minutes before serving.

Garnish with additional chopped parsley if desired, and serve your stuffed mushroom caps as an appetizer or side dish.

Benefits of Stuffed Mushroom Caps:

i. **Rich in Nutrients:** Mushrooms are a good source of vitamins, minerals (like selenium and copper), and antioxidants. They also provide dietary fiber.

ii. **Low in Calories:** Mushrooms are low in calories and make a healthier alternative to traditional appetizers like fried foods.

iii. **Protein:** The breadcrumbs and Parmesan cheese (or vegan alternative) provide a modest amount of protein, making these stuffed mushrooms a satisfying and flavorful option.

iv. **Versatile:** You can customize the stuffing with various ingredients like herbs, different cheeses, garlic, or even cooked vegetables to suit your taste.

v. **Appetizer or Side Dish:** Stuffed mushroom caps can be served as a

> delicious appetizer for parties or as a side dish alongside your main meal.

vi. **Umami Flavor:** Mushrooms have a rich, savory flavor known as umami, which adds depth and complexity to the dish.

vii. **Finger Food:** Stuffed mushroom caps are convenient finger food, making them a popular choice for gatherings and parties.

viii. **Vegetarian/Vegan-Friendly:** This recipe can be easily adapted to be vegetarian or vegan by choosing suitable cheese alternatives and breadcrumbs.

ix. **Gluten-Free Option:** Use gluten-free breadcrumbs to make this dish suitable for those with gluten sensitivities or allergies.

Stuffed mushroom caps are not only tasty but also provide a nutritious and satisfying appetizer or side dish option. They are a great way to incorporate more vegetables into your diet while indulging in a delightful treat.

2. Crispy Avocado Bites:

Creamy avocado slices, coated in a crunchy breadcrumb and seasoning mix, are fried to a golden crisp. The result is a delectable fusion of textures – creamy on the inside and crispy on the outside. Dip these bites into a tangy vegan aioli or salsa for an appetizer that's sure to disappear as soon as it hits the table.

How to Prepare:

Ingredients:

i. 2 ripe avocados, sliced into bite-sized pieces
ii. 1 cup panko breadcrumbs
iii. 1/2 cup all-purpose flour (or a gluten-free alternative)
iv. 2 large eggs (or flaxseed eggs for a vegan option)
v. 1 teaspoon paprika
vi. 1/2 teaspoon garlic powder
vii. 1/2 teaspoon onion powder
viii. Salt and black pepper to taste
ix. Cooking spray or vegetable oil for frying

Optional: dipping sauce (e.g., sriracha mayo, ranch dressing, or salsa)

Instructions:

i. In a shallow bowl, combine the panko breadcrumbs, paprika, garlic powder, onion powder, salt, and black pepper. Mix well to create a seasoned breadcrumb mixture.
ii. In another shallow bowl, place the all-purpose flour.

<ol type="i" start="3">
<li>In a third shallow bowl, whisk the eggs (or prepare flaxseed eggs by mixing 2 tablespoons of ground flaxseed with 6 tablespoons of water and letting it sit for a few minutes until it thickens).</li>
<li>Take each avocado slice and coat it first in the flour, shaking off any excess, then dip it into the beaten egg (or flaxseed egg), and finally, coat it with the seasoned breadcrumb mixture, ensuring it's well coated. Place the coated avocado pieces on a plate or tray.</li>
<li>Heat a skillet or frying pan over medium-high heat and add enough cooking spray or vegetable oil to cover the bottom of the pan.</li>
<li>Once the oil is hot, carefully add the breaded avocado pieces in a single layer, making sure not to overcrowd the pan. Fry them for about 2-3 minutes per side or until they are golden brown and crispy. You may need to do this in batches.</li>
<li>Remove the crispy avocado bites from the pan and place them on a plate lined with paper towels to drain any excess oil.</li>
<li>Serve the crispy avocado bites hot with your choice of dipping sauce.</li>
</ol>

Benefits of Crispy Avocado Bites:

i. **Avocado Nutrition:** Avocado is a nutrient-dense fruit that provides healthy monounsaturated fats, fiber, vitamins (like folate, vitamin K, and vitamin C), minerals (potassium and magnesium), and antioxidants.

ii. **Fiber:** Avocado is a good source of dietary fiber, which aids in digestion and helps you feel fuller for longer.

iii. **Vegan/Vegetarian Option:** By using flaxseed eggs instead of traditional eggs, this recipe can be made vegan, making it suitable for those following a plant-based diet.

iv. **Protein:** The combination of eggs (or flaxseed eggs) and breadcrumbs provides a modest amount of protein, making these bites more satisfying.

v. **Gluten-Free Option:** You can easily make this recipe gluten-free by using gluten-free flour and breadcrumbs.

vi. **Customizable:** You can adapt the seasoning and dipping sauce to your taste, making this dish versatile and suitable for different preferences.

vii. **Delicious Appetizer or Snack:** Crispy avocado bites are a flavorful and satisfying appetizer, party snack, or game-day treat.

viii. **Healthy Fats:** Avocado is known for its heart-healthy monounsaturated fats, which can support overall cardiovascular health.

ix. **Quick and Easy:** This recipe is relatively simple and quick to prepare, making it a convenient option for busy days or when you need a tasty snack.

Enjoy these crispy avocado bites as a delightful appetizer or snack that combines the creamy richness of avocado with a crispy, seasoned coating. They're not only delicious but also offer a range of health benefits.

3. Zesty Buffalo Cauliflower Wings:

Buffalo wings go vegan in this spicy and tangy cauliflower rendition. Bite-sized cauliflower florets are battered and baked to perfection, then tossed in a lip-smacking buffalo sauce. Serve them with celery sticks and vegan ranch dressing for a fiery, finger-licking appetizer that's perfect for game nights or parties.

How to Prepare:

Ingredients:

For the Cauliflower:

i. Cut 1 head of cauliflower into florets
ii. 1 cup all-purpose flour (or chickpea flour for a gluten-free option)
iii. 1 cup water
iv. 1 teaspoon garlic powder
v. 1/2 teaspoon paprika
vi. Salt and black pepper to taste

For the Buffalo Sauce:

i. 1/2 cup hot sauce (such as Frank's RedHot or your favorite brand)
ii. 1/4 cup melted vegan butter (or regular butter if not following a vegan diet)
iii. 1 tablespoon white vinegar
iv. 1/2 teaspoon garlic powder
v. 1/2 teaspoon cayenne pepper (adjust to taste)
vi. Salt to taste

Instructions:

For the Cauliflower:

i. Heat oven temperature to 450°F (232°C). then line a baking sheet with parchment paper or lightly grease it.
ii. In a mixing bowl, combine the flour, water, garlic powder, paprika, salt, and

> black pepper. Mix until you have a smooth batter.

iii. Dip each cauliflower floret into the batter, ensuring it's coated evenly. Allow any excess batter to drip off.

iv. Place the coated cauliflower florets on the prepared baking sheet, making sure they are spaced out and not touching each other.

v. Bake in the preheated oven for 20-25 minutes or until the cauliflower is tender and the batter becomes crispy and golden brown. You may need to flip the florets halfway through for even cooking.

For the Buffalo Sauce:

i. While the cauliflower is baking, prepare the Buffalo sauce. In a small saucepan over low heat, combine the hot sauce, melted vegan butter (or regular butter), white vinegar, garlic powder, cayenne pepper, and salt.

ii. Heat the sauce gently, stirring until well combined and heated through. Taste and adjust the seasoning if needed.

iii. Remove the sauce from heat and set it aside.

Assembly:

i. Once the cauliflower is done baking, transfer the hot cauliflower florets to a mixing bowl.

ii. Pour the prepared Buffalo sauce over the cauliflower and toss until the florets are evenly coated with the sauce.

iii. Serve the zesty Buffalo cauliflower wings immediately with your choice of dipping sauce and celery sticks.

Benefits of Zesty Buffalo Cauliflower Wings:

i. **Vegan/Vegetarian-Friendly:** This recipe uses cauliflower instead of chicken, making it a vegan or vegetarian alternative to traditional Buffalo wings.

ii. **Lower in Calories and Fat:** Compared to traditional deep-fried chicken wings, cauliflower wings are typically lower in calories and saturated fat, making them a healthier choice.

iii. **Rich in Fiber and Vitamins:** Cauliflower is a good source of dietary fiber, vitamins (like vitamin C and vitamin K), and minerals (such as potassium and folate).

iv. **Gluten-Free Option:** By using chickpea flour instead of all-purpose flour, you can make this recipe gluten-free, suitable for those with gluten sensitivities or allergies.

v. **Customizable Heat:** You can adjust the level of spiciness by varying the amount of cayenne pepper in the Buffalo sauce.

vi. **Flavorful Snack or Appetizer:** Zesty Buffalo cauliflower wings are a flavorful and satisfying snack or appetizer for parties, game days, or gatherings.

vii. **Quick and Easy:** This recipe is relatively quick and straightforward to prepare, making it a convenient option for a tasty treat.

viii. **Versatile:** You can customize the sauce and seasonings to your taste preferences, allowing for a variety of flavor combinations.

Enjoy these zesty Buffalo cauliflower wings as a delicious and healthier alternative to traditional Buffalo wings. They provide a satisfying and flavorful snack while incorporating the benefits of cauliflower and a lower calorie and fat content.

4. Spinach and Artichoke Dip:

Creamy, cheesy, and utterly irresistible – this spinach and artichoke dip is a crowd-pleaser. A blend of cashews, nutritional yeast, and spices creates a creamy base, while spinach and artichokes add a burst of flavor and nutrition. Bake until bubbly and serve with crispy tortilla chips or toasted baguette slices for a comforting appetizer.

How to Prepare:

Ingredients:

i. 1 (10-ounce) package of frozen chopped spinach, thawed and drained

ii. 1 (14-ounce) can artichoke hearts, drained and chopped

iii. 1 cup grated Parmesan cheese (or a vegan alternative)

iv. 1 cup mayonnaise (or a vegan mayo)

v. 1 cup sour cream (or a dairy-free sour cream)

vi. 1 cup shredded mozzarella cheese (or a vegan mozzarella)

vii. 3 cloves garlic, minced

viii. Salt and black pepper to taste

Optional: Red pepper flakes for a bit of heat

Tortilla chips, bread, or vegetable sticks for dipping

Instructions:

i. Preheat your oven to 375°F (190°C).

ii. In a large mixing bowl, combine the chopped spinach, chopped artichoke hearts, grated Parmesan cheese, mayonnaise, sour cream, shredded mozzarella cheese, minced garlic, and optional red pepper flakes. Mix everything until well combined.

iii. Use black pepper and salt to the mixture as seasoning, (to taste). Be cautious with the salt, as some of the cheeses may already be salty.

iv. Transfer the spinach and artichoke dip mixture to an ovenproof baking dish.

v. Bake in the preheated oven for approximately 25-30 minutes or until the dip is hot, bubbly, and lightly browned on top.

vi. Remove from the oven and let it cool for a few minutes before serving.

vii. Serve your spinach and artichoke dip with tortilla chips, slices of baguette, pita bread, or vegetable sticks for dipping.

Benefits of Spinach and Artichoke Dip:

i. **Nutrient-Rich Ingredients:** Spinach and artichokes are both nutrient-dense vegetables. Spinach is rich in vitamins (A, C, K, and folate), minerals (iron and calcium), and antioxidants. Artichokes are a good source of dietary fiber, vitamin C, and potassium.

ii. **Protein and Calcium:** Dairy-based versions of this dip contain protein and calcium from the cheeses, sour cream, and mayonnaise.

iii. **Vegan and Dairy-Free Options:** You can easily make this dip vegan or dairy-free by using plant-based cheeses, vegan mayonnaise, and dairy-free sour cream.

iv. **Flavorful Appetizer:** Spinach and artichoke dip is a flavorful and creamy appetizer that is popular at parties, gatherings, and potlucks.

v. **Versatile:** This dip can be served with a variety of dippers, including tortilla chips, bread, crackers, or vegetable sticks, making it a versatile party favorite.

vi. **Fiber-Rich:** The combination of spinach and artichokes adds dietary fiber to the dip, which can support digestive health.

vii. **Homemade:** Making this dip at home allows you to control the ingredients and customize it to your taste preferences, including adjusting the level of garlic or spice.

viii. **Warm and Comforting:** This dip is served warm and is a comforting and indulgent treat, perfect for sharing with friends and family.

While spinach and artichoke dip is a delicious treat, it's important to enjoy it in moderation, as it can be high in calories, fats, and sodium, especially if made with dairy-based ingredients. However, it provides a flavorful way to incorporate nutrient-rich vegetables into your diet and is a crowd-pleaser at social gatherings.

5. **Veggie Sushi Rolls**:

Get creative in the kitchen by crafting your vegan sushi rolls. Nori seaweed sheets envelop a colorful assortment of fresh veggies, avocado, and tofu. Serve with soy sauce, wasabi, and pickled ginger for an authentic sushi experience right at home.

How to Prepare:

Ingredients:

For the Sushi Rice:

 i. 1 cup sushi rice (short-grain white rice)
 ii. 2 cups water
 iii. 1/4 cup rice vinegar
 iv. 2 tablespoons sugar
 v. 1 teaspoon salt

For the Veggie Filling (Customizable):

 i. 1 cucumber, thinly sliced into strips
 ii. 1 carrot, thinly sliced into strips or julienned
 iii. 1 avocado, sliced

iv.   1 bell pepper, thinly sliced into strips

v.   1/2 cup thinly sliced red cabbage (optional, for color and crunch)

vi.   10-12 sheets of nori (seaweed) wrappers

vii.   Soy sauce, wasabi, and pickled ginger for serving

Equipment:

i.   Bamboo sushi rolling mat (makisu)

ii.   Plastic wrap or a large, resealable plastic bag

iii.   Sharp knife for slicing the sushi rolls

Instructions:

For the Sushi Rice:

i.   Rinse the sushi rice in a fine-mesh strainer under cold running water until the water runs clear. Drain thoroughly.

ii.   Using a saucepan of medium size, combine the rinsed rice and water. Over a high heat, bring to a boil. Once it boils, reduce the heat to low, cover, and simmer for about 18-20 minutes, or until the rice is tender and the water is absorbed.

iii.   While the rice is cooking, in a small saucepan, combine the rice vinegar, sugar, and salt. Heat over low heat, stirring until the sugar and salt dissolve. Remove from heat and let it cool.

iv. Once the rice is cooked, transfer it to a large bowl and let it cool slightly. Gradually add the vinegar mixture, gently folding it into the rice with a wooden or plastic spatula. Be careful not to overmix; you want the rice to be sticky but not mushy.

For Assembling the Sushi Rolls:

i. Lay a bamboo sushi rolling mat on a clean surface and cover it with plastic wrap or a large resealable plastic bag. This prevents the rice from sticking to the mat.

ii. Place a sheet of nori, shiny side down, on the mat.

iii. Wet your fingers to prevent sticking, and take about a handful of sushi rice. Spread it evenly over the nori, leaving about 1/2 inch of nori uncovered at the top edge.

iv. Arrange your choice of vegetable fillings in a horizontal line in the center of the rice-covered nori.

v. Lift the edge of the bamboo mat closest to you and begin rolling it away from you, tucking in the fillings as you go. Apply gentle pressure to create a tight roll.

vi. Wet the exposed edge of the nori with a bit of water and press to seal the roll.

vii. Use a sharp knife dipped in water to slice the sushi roll into bite-sized pieces. Clean the knife between cuts for clean edges.

viii. Repeat the process with the remaining nori sheets and fillings.

ix. Serve your veggie sushi rolls with soy sauce, wasabi, and pickled ginger.

Benefits of Veggie Sushi Rolls:

i. **Nutrient-Rich:** Veggie sushi rolls are packed with vegetables, which provide essential vitamins, minerals, and dietary fiber.

ii. **Low in Calories:** They are relatively low in calories compared to sushi rolls with fish or seafood, making them a lighter and healthier option.

iii. **Vegan/Vegetarian-Friendly:** Veggie sushi rolls are naturally vegetarian and vegan, making them suitable for plant-based diets.

iv. **Customizable:** You can customize the fillings to your liking, adding your favorite vegetables, tofu, or other plant-based ingredients.

v. **Rich in Healthy Fats:** Avocado is a common ingredient in veggie sushi rolls and provides heart-healthy monounsaturated fats.

vi. **Gluten-Free Option:** As long as you use gluten-free soy sauce (tamari) or a gluten-free alternative, these rolls can be made gluten-free.

vii. **Fun and Creative:** Making sushi rolls at home can be a fun and creative culinary experience for individuals or groups.

viii. **Portion Control:** Sushi rolls are typically served in small portions, which can help with portion control and mindful eating.

Veggie sushi rolls are not only delicious but also a nutritious and visually appealing dish. They offer a range of health benefits, making them a popular choice for those looking for a tasty and wholesome meal or snack.

Conclusion:

Chapter 2 is inviting you to elevate your appetizer game with plant-based flair. These recipes not only cater to your taste buds but also cater to your conscience, as they are cruelty-free and environmentally friendly. Whether you're hosting a gathering or simply craving a delightful snack, these Appetizing Appetizers will be the star of the show.

Chapter 3:

Sensational Soups.

As the seasons change and a chill creeps into the air, nothing warms the heart and soul quite like a bowl of comforting soup. In this chapter, we explore Sensational Soups, offering an array of nourishing, flavorful, and entirely plant-based soup recipes that will soothe your senses and leave you craving more.

1. **Classic Tomato Soup**:

Start your soup journey with a timeless favorite. This classic tomato soup combines ripe, juicy tomatoes with aromatic herbs and a hint of sweetness. Silky smooth and satisfying, it's the perfect companion to a grilled vegan cheese sandwich or a crusty baguette for dipping.

How to Prepare:

Ingredients:

i. 2 tablespoons olive oil
ii. 1 onion, chopped
iii. 2 cloves garlic, minced
iv. 1 carrot, peeled and chopped
v. Chop 1 stalk of celery
vi. 1 (28-ounce) can crushed tomatoes
vii. 1 (14-ounce) can diced tomatoes
viii. 4 cups vegetable broth
ix. 1 teaspoon dried basil

x.   Dried oregano, (1 teaspoon)

xi.   1/2 teaspoon dried thyme

xii.   Salt and black pepper to taste

xiii.   1/4 cup fresh basil leaves, chopped (for garnish)

xiv. 1/4 cup heavy cream or coconut cream (optional, for added creaminess)

Instructions:

i.   Heat the olive oil in a large pot over medium heat.

ii.   Add the chopped onion, garlic, carrot, and celery to the pot. Cook for about 5-7 minutes or until the vegetables have softened and the onion is translucent.

iii.   Stir in the crushed tomatoes, diced tomatoes, vegetable broth, dried basil, dried oregano, dried thyme, salt, and black pepper.

iv.   After bringing the mixture to a boil, bring the heat to low. Simmer, covered, for about 20-25 minutes, stirring occasionally.

v.   Using immersion blender, puree the soup until it beomes smooth and creamy. If you don't have an immersion blender, carefully transfer the soup in batches to a regular blender, blend until smooth, and return it to the pot.

vi. If desired, stir in the heavy cream or coconut cream to add creaminess to the soup. Heat the soup for an additional 2-3 minutes over low heat, stirring gently.

vii. Taste and adjust the seasoning, adding more salt and pepper if needed.

viii. Serve the classic tomato soup hot, garnished with chopped fresh basil leaves.

Benefits of Classic Tomato Soup:

i. **Rich in Vitamins and Minerals:** Tomato soup is a good source of vitamins such as vitamin C, vitamin K, and various B vitamins. It also contains minerals like potassium.

ii. **Antioxidants:** Tomatoes are rich in antioxidants, including lycopene, which has been associated with a reduced risk of chronic diseases and may help protect against certain cancers.

iii. **Low in Calories:** Tomato soup is typically low in calories, making it a healthy option for those looking to manage their calorie intake.

iv. **Hydration:** Tomato soup has a high water content, contributing to your daily hydration needs.

v. **Fiber:** The addition of vegetables like carrots and celery provides dietary fiber, which supports digestive health and helps you feel fuller for longer.

vi. **Heart Health:** The lycopene and potassium in tomatoes may contribute to improved heart health by reducing the risk of high blood pressure and heart disease.

vii. **Immune Support:** The vitamin C in tomato soup can help boost your immune system.

viii. **Comfort Food:** Tomato soup is a comforting and soothing dish that can provide emotional comfort during cold or stressful times.

ix. **Easy to Make:** This classic tomato soup recipe is relatively easy to prepare and can be made in under an hour.

x. **Customizable:** You can customize your tomato soup by adding herbs, spices, or additional vegetables to suit your taste preferences.

Classic tomato soup is not only delicious but also a nutritious and comforting dish that offers a range of health benefits. It's a versatile meal that can be enjoyed as a starter, side dish, or even a light main course.

2. **Spicy Thai Coconut Curry:**

Travel to the vibrant streets of Thailand with a rich and aromatic coconut curry soup. Infused with lemongrass, ginger, and red curry paste, this soup boasts a symphony of flavors and textures, including tofu or chickpeas and an assortment of vegetables. Topped with fresh cilantro and a squeeze of lime, it's a taste sensation that'll transport your taste buds.

How to Prepare:

Ingredients:

For the Curry Paste (Alternatively, you can use store-bought Thai red curry paste):

i. 3-4 dried red chilies, soaked in hot water for 15 minutes and drained (adjust for desired heat)

ii. Add 2 cloves of garlic

iii. Chop 1 shallot

iv. 1 lemongrass stalk, sliced (use only the bottom 4-5 inches)

v. 1 thumb-sized piece of fresh ginger, chopped

vi. 1 thumb-sized piece of fresh galangal (or substitute with more ginger), chopped

vii. 1 teaspoon ground coriander

viii. 1/2 teaspoonful of ground cumin

ix. 1/2 teaspoon shrimp paste (skip for vegetarian/vegan)

x.   Zest and juice of 1 lime

xi.   1 tablespoon vegetable oil

For the Curry:

i.   2 tablespoons vegetable oil

ii.   1 onion, finely chopped

iii.   2-3 tablespoons of the homemade curry paste (or store-bought)

iv.   14 ounces of coconut milk (or 1 can)

v.   1 cup vegetable broth

vi.   2 tablespoons soy sauce (or fish sauce for non-vegetarian)

vii.   1 tablespoonful of palm sugar (brown sugar)

viii.   Thinly slice 1 red bell pepper

ix.   1 green bell pepper, thinly sliced

x.   1 zucchini, thinly sliced

xi.   1 carrot, thinly sliced

xii.   Add 1 cup of broccoli florets

xiii.   1 cup firm tofu, cubed (optional)

xiv.   Fresh basil or cilantro leaves for garnish

xv.   Cooked jasmine rice or rice noodles for serving

Instructions:

For the Curry Paste:

i.   Place all the curry paste ingredients in a food processor or blender.

ii.   Blend until you have a smooth paste. You may need to scrape down the sides of the blender or add a little water to help with blending.

For the Curry:

i.   In a large skillet or wok, heat 2 tablespoons of vegetable oil over medium-high heat.

ii.   Add the chopped onion and sauté for 2-3 minutes until it becomes translucent.

iii.   Stir in the homemade curry paste (or store-bought) and cook for 2-3 minutes, allowing the flavors to release and the paste to become fragrant.

iv.   Pour the coconut milk, brown sugar, fish sauce (or soy sauce), vegetable broth. Stir to mix. Then bring the mixture gently to a simmer.

v.   Add the red and green bell peppers, zucchini, carrot, broccoli, and tofu (if using). Simmer for about 5-7 minutes, or until the vegetables are tender and the sauce has thickened slightly. Taste the curry and adjust the seasoning by adding more soy sauce or sugar if needed.

vi.   Serve the spicy Thai coconut curry hot over jasmine rice or rice noodles. You may also garnish with cilantro leaves or fresh basil.

Benefits of Spicy Thai Coconut Curry:

i. **Rich Flavor Profile:** Thai coconut curry is known for its bold and complex flavors, combining spicy, sweet, and savory elements in one dish.

ii. **Vegetarian/Vegan-Friendly:** This recipe can be easily adapted to be vegetarian or vegan by using vegetable broth and omitting shrimp paste and fish sauce, substituting with soy sauce.

iii. **Diverse Vegetables:** Thai coconut curry typically contains an array of colorful vegetables, providing various vitamins, minerals, and dietary fiber.

iv. **Healthy Fats:** Coconut milk in the curry provides healthy fats, which are essential for energy and nutrient absorption.

v. **Protein Source:** You can add tofu, tempeh, or seitan for plant-based protein, or include meat or seafood for additional protein.

vi. **Spices and Herbs:** The spices and herbs used in Thai curry, such as lemongrass, ginger, and galangal, offer potential health benefits, including anti-inflammatory properties.

vii. **Customizable Heat:** You can adjust the level of spiciness by controlling the amount of chili used in the curry paste.

viii. **Comfort Food:** Thai coconut curry is a comforting and satisfying dish, perfect for warming up on cold days or enjoying year-round.

ix. **Rice or Noodles:** You can serve it with jasmine rice or rice noodles, providing flexibility in your meal choice.

Enjoy the delicious flavors and health benefits of this homemade spicy Thai coconut curry. It's a hearty and comforting meal that can be customized to suit your taste preferences and dietary needs.

3. **Hearty Lentil Stew:**

Lentils take center stage in this hearty stew, creating a filling and nutritious meal. The earthy flavors of lentils mingle with carrots, celery, and potatoes, while a blend of herbs and spices adds depth. This stew is perfect for a comforting weeknight dinner or a warm, cozy lunch.

How to Prepare:

Ingredients:

i. 1 cup green or brown lentils, rinsed and drained

ii. 1 onion, chopped

iii.   2 carrots, chopped

iv.   2 celery stalks, chopped

v.   Add 3 cloves of minced garlic

vi.   1 can (14 ounces) diced tomatoes

vii.   4 cups vegetable broth

viii.   2 bay leaves

ix.   1 teaspoon dried thyme

x.   1 teaspoon dried rosemary

xi.   Add black pepper and salt to the taste as you like

xii.   2 tablespoons olive oil

xiii.   2 cups chopped kale or spinach (optional)

xiv.   1 tablespoon balsamic vinegar (optional)

xv.   Fresh parsley or cilantro for garnish (optional)

Instructions:

i.   Using a Dutch oven or a moderately big soup pot over medium-level heat, heat the olive oil.

ii.   Add the chopped onion, carrots, and celery to the pot. Sauté for about 5 minutes until the vegetables begin to soften.

iii.   Stir in the minced garlic and cook for an additional minute until fragrant.

iv.   Add the lentils, diced tomatoes (with their juice), vegetable broth, bay leaves, dried thyme, dried rosemary, salt, and black pepper to the pot. Stir to combine.

v. Let the mixture boil, then bring down the heat to low and cover it. Then simmer until the lentils are tender and the stew has thickened, (say about 25-30 minutes)

vi. If using, add the chopped kale or spinach to the stew during the last 5 minutes of cooking, allowing it to wilt.

vii. Remove the bay leaves from the stew.

viii. Stir in the balsamic vinegar for added flavor (if desired).

ix. Taste the stew and adjust the seasoning with more salt and pepper if needed.

x. Serve the hearty lentil stew hot, garnished with fresh parsley or cilantro if desired.

Benefits of Hearty Lentil Stew:

i. **High in Plant-Based Protein:** Lentils are a fantastic source of plant-based protein, making this stew a satisfying and nutritious option, especially for vegetarians and vegans.

ii. **Rich in Fiber:** Lentils are packed with dietary fiber, which supports digestive health and helps you feel full and satisfied.

iii. **Low in Fat:** This stew is typically low in saturated fats, especially if you use minimal oil for sautéing.

iv. **Nutrient-Dense:** The stew contains an array of vegetables, including carrots, celery, and kale or spinach, which provide vitamins, minerals, and antioxidants.

v. **Heart-Healthy:** Lentils are known for their heart-healthy benefits, as they can help lower cholesterol levels and reduce the risk of heart disease.

vi. **Gluten-Free:** Lentils are naturally gluten-free, making this stew suitable for individuals with gluten sensitivities or celiac disease.

vii. **Easy to Customize:** You can tailor the stew to your preferences by adding different vegetables or herbs and adjusting the seasonings.

viii. **Budget-Friendly:** Lentils are an economical source of protein and nutrients, making this stew a budget-friendly meal option.

ix. **Warm and Comforting:** Hearty lentil stew is a warming and comforting dish, perfect for chilly days or as a comforting meal year-round.

x. **Versatile:** You can serve this stew as a main course or as a side dish. It's also a great option for meal prep and can be stored for future meals.

Enjoy this hearty lentil stew as a wholesome and satisfying meal that provides a range of health benefits while comforting your taste buds. It's a nutritious choice for those looking to incorporate more plant-based protein and fiber into their diet.

4. **Creamy Broccoli Cheddar Soup:**

Indulge in a creamy broccoli cheddar soup without the dairy. Cashews, nutritional yeast, and plant-based milk come together to create a luscious, cheesy base, while tender broccoli florets add a burst of freshness. A dash of nutmeg and a sprinkle of vegan cheddar shreds on top complete this satisfying soup.

Preparation:
Ingredients:

i. Add 4 cups fresh broccoli florets (about 2 small heads)
ii. Chopped onion- 1
iii. Minced garlic- 2 cloves
iv. Vegetable broth- 3 cups
v. 1 cup milk (whole, 2%, or plant-based)
vi. 1/4 cup all-purpose flour (or a gluten-free alternative)

vii.   2 cups shredded sharp cheddar cheese (or a vegan cheddar alternative)

viii.   2 tablespoons butter (or a vegan butter alternative)

ix.   Add black pepper and salt to taste

x.   Garnishes (optional): additional cheddar cheese (shredded), croutons, or fresh chopped parsley

Instructions:

i.   Using a large Dutch oven or pot, melt the butter over medium heat.

ii.   Add the chopped onion and garlic to the pot. Sauté for about 3-4 minutes until the onion becomes translucent.

iii.   Over the sautéed onions and garlic, sprinkle the flour. After stirring well to form a roux, then cook for 2-3 minutes to remove the taste of raw flour.

iv.   While continuously whisking to prevent lumps, pour in the vegetable broth gradually. Bring the mixture to a boil, then reduce the heat to low level.

v.   Add the broccoli florets to the pot and simmer for about 10-15 minutes or until the broccoli is tender while stirring occasionally.

vi.   Using an immersion blender, blend the soup until it's smooth and creamy.

Alternatively, carefully transfer the soup in batches to a blender, blend until smooth, and return it to the pot.

vii. Return the pot to low heat and add the milk. Stir to combine.

viii. Gradually add the shredded cheddar cheese to the soup, stirring until it's fully melted and the soup is creamy.

ix. Season the soup with salt and black pepper to taste.

x. Serve the creamy broccoli cheddar soup hot, garnished with additional shredded cheddar cheese, croutons, or fresh chopped parsley if desired.

Benefits of Creamy Broccoli Cheddar Soup:

i. **Nutrient-Rich:** Broccoli is a nutritional powerhouse, rich in vitamins (C, K), minerals (folate, potassium), and dietary fiber. It's also a source of antioxidants.

ii. **Calcium and Protein:** Cheddar cheese provides calcium and protein, which are essential for bone health and muscle function.

iii. **Versatile:** This soup can be customized to suit various dietary preferences. You can use dairy or plant-based milk, and there are many vegan cheddar cheese alternatives available.

iv. **Vegetarian-Friendly:** The soup is vegetarian, but it can be made vegan by using plant-based milk and vegan cheddar cheese.

v. **Creamy Texture:** The creamy texture of this soup is comforting and satisfying, making it a filling meal or appetizer.

vi. **Comfort Food:** Creamy broccoli cheddar soup is a classic comfort food, perfect for warming up on cold days or enjoying as a cozy meal.

vii. **Easy to Make:** This recipe is relatively easy to prepare and can be ready in under 30 minutes.

viii. **Kid-Friendly:** The combination of creamy cheese and broccoli makes this soup appealing to both adults and children.

ix. **Weight Management:** Broccoli is low in calories and high in fiber, which can support weight management and overall health.

x. **Budget-Friendly:** This soup is cost-effective and can be made with simple, affordable ingredients.

Enjoy the rich and comforting flavors of creamy broccoli cheddar soup, which combines the nutritional benefits of broccoli with the creamy indulgence of cheddar cheese. It's a satisfying and flavorful dish suitable for various dietary preferences.

5. **Tortilla Soup with Avocado:**

Enjoy the vibrant flavors of Mexican cuisine with a zesty tortilla soup. This dish features a tomato-based broth infused with chili spices, corn, black beans, and topped with crispy tortilla strips, creamy avocado slices, and a squeeze of lime. It's a bowl of comfort with a spicy kick.

How to Prepare:

Ingredients:

For the Soup:

i.   1 tablespoon olive oil
ii.   1 onion, chopped
iii.   2 cloves garlic, minced
iv.   1 jalapeño pepper, seeds removed and finely chopped (adjust for desired heat)
v.   1 red bell pepper, chopped
vi.   1 yellow bell pepper, chopped
vii.   1 can (14 ounces) diced tomatoes
viii.   14 ounces (1 can) of black beans. drain and rinse
ix.   14 ounces (1 can) of corn kernels, (drained)
x.   4 cups vegetable broth

xi. 1 teaspoon ground cumin
xii. 1 teaspoon chili powder (adjust to taste)
xiii. Add black pepper and salt to taste
xiv. Juice of 1 lime

For Garnish:

i. 2 avocados, diced
ii. Tortilla chips or strips
iii. Fresh cilantro leaves, chopped
iv. Shredded cheese (cheddar, Monterey Jack, or a vegan alternative)
v. Sour cream or dairy-free yogurt (optional)

Instructions:

i. In a large soup pot or Dutch oven, heat the olive oil over medium heat.
ii. Add the chopped onion, garlic, and jalapeño to the pot. Sauté for about 3-4 minutes until the onion becomes translucent and the mixture is fragrant.
iii. Stir in the chopped red and yellow bell peppers and cook for an additional 3-4 minutes until they begin to soften.
iv. Add the diced tomatoes, black beans, corn, vegetable broth, ground cumin, and chili powder to the pot. Season with salt and black pepper to taste. Stir to combine.
v. Let the soup to boil, then rbring the heat to low. Cover and simmer for about 15-20

minutes, allowing the flavors to meld together.

vi. Stir in the lime juice and taste the soup. Adjust the seasoning with more salt, black pepper, or chili powder if needed.

vii. To serve, ladle the tortilla soup into bowls. Top each bowl with diced avocado, tortilla chips or strips, chopped cilantro, and shredded cheese.

Optionally, add a dollop of sour cream or dairy-free yogurt for extra creaminess.

Benefits of Tortilla Soup with Avocado:

i. **Rich in Fiber:** This soup contains black beans and corn, both of which are excellent sources of dietary fiber. Fiber supports digestive health and helps keep you feeling full.

ii. **Vitamins and Minerals:** The bell peppers and tomatoes in the soup provide vitamins (A, C) and minerals (folate, potassium).

iii. **Healthy Fats:** Avocado is a nutritious addition that contributes heart-healthy monounsaturated fats.

iv. **Protein:** Black beans are a good source of plant-based protein, making this soup satisfying.

v. **Antioxidants:** The combination of vegetables in the soup offers a variety of antioxidants, which can help protect your cells from oxidative damage.

vi. **Customizable Heat:** You can adjust the level of spiciness by varying the amount of jalapeño or chili powder used in the soup.

vii. **Versatile:** Tortilla soup can be made with various toppings, allowing for customization based on your preferences.

viii. **Taste and Texture:** The combination of flavors and textures, including the creamy avocado, crunchy tortilla chips, and savory broth, makes this soup both delicious and satisfying.

ix. **Quick and Easy:** This soup is relatively quick and easy to prepare, making it a convenient option for a tasty meal.

Enjoy the flavors and health benefits of tortilla soup with avocado. It's a nutritious and satisfying dish that combines the richness of avocado with the heartiness of black beans and the flavors of a warm, comforting soup.

Chapter 4:

Savory Salads.

Chapter 4 will take us on a journey into the world of Savory Salads – a culinary adventure where vibrant vegetables, fresh herbs, and zesty dressings come together to create mouthwatering, satisfying, and entirely vegan salads. These recipes prove that salads are far from boring and can be the star of your meal.

1. **Quinoa and Roasted Vegetable Salad:**

Elevate your salad game with this colorful and protein-packed dish. Roasted vegetables like bell peppers, zucchini, and cherry tomatoes mingle with fluffy quinoa, fresh herbs, and a tangy lemon vinaigrette. This salad is a burst of flavors and textures, perfect as a light lunch or a hearty side dish.

How to Prepare:

Ingredients:

For the Salad:

i. Rinse and drain 1 cup of quinoa
ii. 2 cups water or vegetable broth
iii. 2 cups mixed vegetables (such as bell peppers, zucchini, cherry tomatoes, and red onion), chopped into bite-sized pieces

iv.   2 tablespoons olive oil
v.   Salt and black pepper to taste
vi.   1/2 cup fresh spinach or arugula leaves (optional)
vii.   1/4 cup fresh basil or parsley leaves, chopped (optional)

For the Dressing:

i.   3 tablespoons olive oil
ii.   2 tablespoons balsamic vinegar
iii.   1 clove garlic, minced
iv.   1 teaspoon Dijon mustard
v.   Salt and black pepper to taste

Instructions:

For Roasting the Vegetables:

i.   Preheat your oven to 425°F (220°C).
ii.   Place the chopped mixed vegetables on a baking sheet. Drizzle with 2 tablespoons of olive oil, and season with salt and black pepper to taste. Toss to coat evenly.
iii.   Roast the vegetables in the preheated oven for 20-25 minutes, or until they are tender and slightly caramelized. Stir them once or twice during roasting to ensure even cooking.
iv.   Remove the roasted vegetables from the oven and let them cool slightly.

For Cooking the Quinoa:

i. In a medium saucepan, combine the rinsed quinoa and water or vegetable broth. Bring to a boil over high heat.

ii. Once it boils, reduce the heat to low, cover the saucepan, and simmer for about 15 minutes, or until the quinoa is cooked and the liquid is absorbed.

iii. After removing the saucepan from the heat, allow it to sit while covered, for 5 minutes. Then, with a fork, fluff the quinoa. Let it cool down to room temperature.

For the Dressing:

i. In a small bowl, whisk together the olive oil, balsamic vinegar, minced garlic, Dijon mustard, salt, and black pepper.

Assembling the Salad:

i. In a large mixing bowl, combine the cooked quinoa and roasted vegetables.

ii. If desired, add fresh spinach or arugula leaves for extra greens and chopped fresh basil or parsley for added flavor.

iii. Drizzle the dressing over the salad and toss everything together until well combined.

iv. Taste and adjust the seasoning with more salt and black pepper if needed.

v. Serve the quinoa and roasted vegetable salad either warm or at room temperature.

Benefits of Quinoa and Roasted Vegetable Salad:

i. **Protein-Rich:** Quinoa is a complete protein source, containing all nine essential amino acids, making this salad a satisfying and nutritious meal.

ii. **Rich in Fiber:** Quinoa and vegetables provide dietary fiber, which supports digestive health and helps maintain a feeling of fullness.

iii. **Vitamins and Minerals:** The mixed vegetables in the salad contribute vitamins (A, C) and minerals (folate, potassium), enhancing its nutritional value.

iv. **Healthy Fats:** Olive oil in the dressing adds healthy monounsaturated fats, which are beneficial for heart health.

v. **Antioxidants:** The variety of colorful vegetables in the salad offers a range of antioxidants, which can help protect your cells from damage caused by free radicals.

vi. **Customizable:** You can adapt this salad to your preferences by using your favorite vegetables and herbs.

vii. **Vegetarian/Vegan-Friendly:** This salad is naturally vegetarian and vegan, making it suitable for various dietary preferences.

viii. **Low in Saturated Fat:** The salad is low in saturated fats, making it a heart-healthy option.

ix. **Quick and Easy:** Quinoa and roasted vegetable salad is relatively quick and easy to prepare, making it a convenient choice for a wholesome meal.

Enjoy the delicious flavors and health benefits of this quinoa and roasted vegetable salad, which offers a balanced combination of protein, fiber, vitamins, and minerals. It's a versatile dish that can be customized to suit your taste and dietary preferences.

2. Fresh Mediterranean Bowl:

Transport yourself to the shores of the Mediterranean with this fresh and vibrant salad bowl. Cucumber, cherry tomatoes, olives, and red onion are tossed with a lemony tahini dressing and served over a bed of quinoa or couscous. Top it off with crumbled vegan feta and a sprinkle of fresh mint for a taste of the Mediterranean.

How to Prepare:

Ingredients:

For the Bowl:

i.   1 cup cooked quinoa or bulgur wheat (prepared according to package instructions)
ii.   1 cup chickpeas, cooked or canned (drained and rinsed)
iii.   1/2 cup of cherry tomatoes
iv.   1 cucumber, diced
v.   1/2 cup red onion, finely chopped
vi.   1/2 cup Kalamata olives, pitted and sliced
vii.   1/2 cup crumbled feta cheese (optional, omit for a vegan version)
viii. Fresh parsley or cilantro leaves for garnish

For the Dressing:

i.   Extra-virgin olive oil- 3 tablespoons
ii.   2 tablespoons lemon juice
iii.   1 clove garlic, minced
iv.   Dried oregano- 1 teaspoon
v.   Salt and black pepper to taste

Instructions:

For the Dressing:

i.   In a small bowl, whisk together the extra-virgin olive oil, lemon juice, minced garlic, dried oregano, salt, and black pepper. Set aside.

Assembling the Mediterranean Bowl:

i. In a large serving bowl, start with a base of cooked quinoa or bulgur wheat.

ii. Arrange the chickpeas, halved cherry tomatoes, diced cucumber, chopped red onion, and sliced Kalamata olives on top of the quinoa or bulgur wheat.

iii. If using, sprinkle crumbled feta cheese over the bowl.

iv. Drizzle the prepared dressing evenly over the ingredients in the bowl.

v. Garnish the Mediterranean bowl with fresh parsley or cilantro leaves for a burst of freshness.

vi. Toss the salad gently just before serving to ensure the dressing is evenly distributed.

vii. Serve the fresh Mediterranean bowl immediately and enjoy!

Benefits of a Fresh Mediterranean Bowl:

i. **Rich in Nutrients:** A Mediterranean bowl is packed with a variety of nutrient-rich ingredients, including vegetables, whole grains, legumes, and healthy fats.

ii. **Plant-Based Protein:** Chickpeas are a great source of plant-based protein, providing essential amino acids.

iii. **Dietary Fiber:** The combination of vegetables, grains, and legumes in this bowl offers a significant amount of dietary fiber, which supports digestive health and helps with satiety.

iv. **Healthy Fats:** Olive oil and olives are sources of heart-healthy monounsaturated fats, which are a staple of the Mediterranean diet.

v. **Antioxidants:** The colorful vegetables and olives in this bowl provide a range of antioxidants, which help protect cells from oxidative stress.

vi. **Vitamins and Minerals:** Cherry tomatoes, cucumbers, and onions contribute essential vitamins (C, K) and minerals (potassium) to the dish.

vii. **Customizable:** You can customize this bowl with your favorite Mediterranean ingredients, such as roasted red peppers, artichoke hearts, or even grilled chicken or tofu for added protein.

viii. **Flavorful Dressing:** The lemon, garlic, and oregano dressing adds bright and zesty flavors to the bowl.

ix. **Versatile:** A Mediterranean bowl can be enjoyed as a satisfying lunch or dinner option, and you can prepare it in advance for meal prep.

x. **Heart-Healthy:** The Mediterranean diet has been associated with various health benefits, including improved heart health and reduced risk of chronic diseases.

Enjoy the vibrant flavors and health benefits of a fresh Mediterranean bowl, which offers a balance of nutrients, textures, and tastes. It's a versatile and delicious way to incorporate the Mediterranean diet's principles into your meals.

3. Spinach and Strawberry Salad:

Indulge in the delightful combination of sweet and savory with this spinach and strawberry salad. Fresh spinach leaves are adorned with ripe strawberries, candied pecans, and a balsamic vinaigrette that marries all the flavors together perfectly. It's a beautiful and refreshing salad that's perfect for warm weather.

How to Prepare:

Ingredients:

For the Salad:

i. 4 cups fresh baby spinach leaves, washed and dried
ii. 1 1/2 cups fresh strawberries, hulled and sliced
iii. 1/2 cup red onion, thinly sliced

iv. 1/4 cup crumbled feta cheese (optional, omit for a vegan version)
v. 1/4 cup sliced almonds, toasted
vi. Fresh mint leaves for garnish (optional)

For the Dressing:

I. Extra-virgin olive oil- 3 tablespoons
II. 2 tablespoons balsamic vinegar
III. 1 tablespoon honey or maple syrup (for a vegan version)
IV. Add black pepper and salt to your taste

Instructions:

For the Dressing:

i. In a small bowl, whisk together the extra-virgin olive oil, balsamic vinegar, honey or maple syrup (if using), salt, and black pepper. Set aside.

Assembling the Spinach and Strawberry Salad:

i. In a large salad bowl, place the fresh baby spinach leaves.
ii. Arrange the sliced strawberries and thinly sliced red onion on top of the spinach.
iii. If using, sprinkle crumbled feta cheese and toasted sliced almonds over the salad ingredients.

iv. Drizzle the prepared dressing evenly over the salad.

v. Garnish the spinach and strawberry salad with fresh mint leaves for an extra burst of flavor and freshness.

vi. Toss the salad gently just before serving to ensure the dressing is evenly distributed.

vii. Serve the spinach and strawberry salad immediately and enjoy!

Benefits of Spinach and Strawberry Salad:

i. **Nutrient-Rich:** This salad is packed with a variety of nutrients, including vitamins (A, C, K), minerals (potassium, folate), and dietary fiber.

ii. **Antioxidants:** Strawberries are rich in antioxidants, such as vitamin C and anthocyanins, which help protect your cells from oxidative damage.

iii. **Heart-Healthy:** The combination of spinach and strawberries, along with the heart-healthy fats from olive oil and almonds, can support cardiovascular health.

iv. **Dietary Fiber:** Spinach and strawberries are good sources of dietary fiber, which aids digestion and helps you feel full and satisfied.

v. **Protein and Healthy Fats:** Almonds provide plant-based protein and healthy monounsaturated fats, which can help with satiety.

vi. **Low in Calories:** This salad is relatively low in calories, making it a great choice for those looking to manage their calorie intake.

vii. **Customizable:** You can customize the salad by adding other ingredients like grilled chicken, tofu, or avocado for added protein or creaminess.

viii. **Vibrant Flavors:** The combination of sweet strawberries, creamy feta cheese (if used), and the tangy balsamic dressing creates a delightful balance of flavors.

ix. **Refreshing:** The addition of mint leaves adds a refreshing and aromatic element to the salad.

x. **Vegan Option:** You can easily make this salad vegan by omitting the feta cheese and using maple syrup instead of honey in the dressing.

Enjoy the fresh and vibrant flavors of a spinach and strawberry salad, which offers a range of health benefits while delighting your taste buds. It's a perfect choice for a light and nutritious meal or as a side dish for various occasions.

4. **Rainbow Coleslaw with Creamy Dressing**:

Brighten up your table with this colorful and crunchy coleslaw. A medley of shredded cabbage, carrots, bell peppers, and red onion is combined with a creamy and tangy dressing. This salad is a staple at picnics, barbecues, or as a side dish to your favorite plant-based burgers and sandwiches.

How to Prepare:

Ingredients:

For the Coleslaw:

i. 4 cups thinly sliced green cabbage
ii. 1 cup thinly sliced red cabbage
iii. 1 cup shredded carrots
iv. 1 cup thinly sliced bell peppers (a mix of red, yellow, and green)
v. 1/2 cup thinly sliced red onion
vi. 1/2 cup chopped fresh cilantro or parsley (optional)
vii. 1/4 cup roasted sunflower seeds (optional)

For the Creamy Dressing:

i. 1/2 cup mayonnaise (regular or vegan)
ii. 1/4 cup plain Greek yogurt (or dairy-free yogurt for a vegan version)
iii. Apple cider vinegar- 2 teaspoons

iv. 1 tablespoon honey or maple syrup (for a vegan version)

v. 1 teaspoon Dijon mustard

vi. Salt and black pepper to taste

Instructions:

For the Creamy Dressing:

i. In a small bowl, whisk together the mayonnaise, Greek yogurt, apple cider vinegar, honey or maple syrup (if using), Dijon mustard, salt, and black pepper. Season, taste and adjust as needed. Then set aside.

Assembling the Rainbow Coleslaw:

i. In a large mixing bowl, combine the thinly sliced green cabbage, red cabbage, shredded carrots, sliced bell peppers, and red onion.

ii. If using, add the chopped fresh cilantro or parsley to the bowl.

iii. Drizzle the creamy dressing over the coleslaw ingredients.

iv. Toss everything together until the vegetables are evenly coated with the dressing.

v. If desired, sprinkle roasted sunflower seeds over the coleslaw for added crunch and flavor.

vi. Refrigerate the rainbow coleslaw for at least 30 minutes before serving to allow the flavors to meld together.

vii. Serve the coleslaw as a refreshing side dish or as a topping for sandwiches, burgers, or tacos.

Benefits of Rainbow Coleslaw with Creamy Dressing:

i. **Rich in Vegetables:** This coleslaw is packed with a variety of colorful vegetables, providing a wide range of vitamins, minerals, and antioxidants.

ii. **Fiber:** Cabbage and carrots are good sources of dietary fiber, which supports digestive health and helps maintain a feeling of fullness.

iii. **Low in Calories:** Coleslaw is typically low in calories, making it a great addition to a balanced diet.

iv. **Protein and Probiotics:** The creamy dressing includes Greek yogurt, which adds protein and probiotics, promoting gut health.

v. **Heart-Healthy Fats:** The inclusion of sunflower seeds provides healthy fats, particularly monounsaturated and polyunsaturated fats.

vi. **Customizable:** You can customize the coleslaw by adding other ingredients like sliced apples, raisins, or dried cranberries for sweetness or sliced almonds for extra crunch.

vii. **Versatile:** This coleslaw can be served on its own as a side dish, as a topping for various sandwiches, or as a complement to grilled dishes.

viii. **Creamy and Tangy:** The creamy dressing adds a rich and tangy flavor to the coleslaw, making it both delicious and satisfying.

ix. **Vegan Option:** You can easily make this coleslaw vegan by using vegan mayonnaise and dairy-free yogurt in the dressing.

x. **Make-Ahead:** Coleslaw can be made in advance and refrigerated, allowing for easy meal prep and planning.

Enjoy the refreshing and nutritious flavors of rainbow coleslaw with creamy dressing. It's a versatile and colorful dish that complements a wide range of meals and provides a boost of essential nutrients.

5. **Caesar Salad with Vegan Caesar Dressing:**

Classic meets vegan in this Caesar salad with a dairy-free twist. Crispy romaine lettuce is tossed with homemade croutons, vegan Caesar dressing, and a sprinkle of vegan parmesan cheese. It's a satisfying and familiar salad that retains all the flavors you love without the need for animal products.

How to Prepare:

Ingredients:

For the Salad:

i.   1 head of romaine lettuce, washed and chopped
ii. 1 cup croutons (store-bought or homemade)
iii. 1/4 cup vegan Parmesan cheese (store-bought or homemade)
iv. Lemon wedges for garnish (optional)

For the Vegan Caesar Dressing:

i.   1/2 cup vegan mayonnaise
ii.   2 tablespoons lemon juice (about 1 lemon)
iii. Cloves of minced garlic- 1-2
iv.   1 teaspoon Dijon mustard
v.   1 teaspoon capers, chopped
vi.   1 teaspoon caper brine (liquid from the caper jar)
vii. 1/2 teaspoon vegan Worcestershire sauce

viii.   Black pepper (ground)- ¼ teaspoon

ix.   Salt to taste

Instructions:

For the Vegan Caesar Dressing:

i.   In a small bowl, whisk together the vegan mayonnaise, lemon juice, minced garlic, Dijon mustard, chopped capers, caper brine, vegan Worcestershire sauce, black pepper, and a pinch of salt.

ii.   Taste the dressing and adjust the seasonings, adding more lemon juice, salt, or pepper as needed. Keep in mind that Caesar dressing should have a tangy and slightly salty flavor.

iii.   Refrigerate the dressing for at least 30 minutes to allow the flavors to meld together.

Assembling the Caesar Salad:

i.   In a large salad bowl, place the washed and chopped romaine lettuce.

ii.   Drizzle the vegan Caesar dressing over the lettuce. Start with a portion of the dressing and add more as needed, as personal preferences for dressing amounts can vary.

iii. Toss the lettuce and dressing together until the lettuce is evenly coated.

iv. Add the croutons to the salad and toss again to combine.

v. Sprinkle the vegan Parmesan cheese over the top of the salad.

vi. **Optionally**, garnish with lemon wedges for an extra burst of freshness.

vii. Serve the Caesar salad immediately as an appetizer, side dish, or main course.

Benefits of Caesar Salad with Vegan Caesar Dressing:

i. **Low in Calories:** Caesar salad is typically lower in calories compared to many other salads, making it a light and satisfying option.

ii. **Vegan-Friendly:** This vegan Caesar salad uses plant-based ingredients, including vegan mayonnaise and Parmesan cheese, making it suitable for vegans and those with dairy allergies.

iii. **Leafy Greens:** Romaine lettuce is a good source of vitamins (A, K, C) and dietary fiber, promoting overall health.

iv. **Protein:** The croutons in the salad provide carbohydrates and some protein, while the dressing can also add a creaminess and richness to the dish.

v. **Flavorful Dressing:** The vegan Caesar dressing combines tangy, savory, and slightly briny flavors, making the salad delicious and satisfying.

vi. **Customizable:** You can customize your Caesar salad by adding ingredients like grilled tofu, chickpeas, or vegan bacon for extra protein and flavor.

vii. **Crunchy Croutons:** Croutons add a delightful crunch to the salad, creating a contrast in textures.

viii. **Make-Ahead:** You can prepare the dressing in advance and store it in the refrigerator, making it convenient for quick salads.

ix. **Suitable for Special Diets:** This salad is suitable for people with various dietary preferences and restrictions, including vegans, vegetarians, and those following a dairy-free diet.

x. **Quick and Easy:** Caesar salad is simple to prepare and can be ready in minutes, making it a convenient option for busy days.

Enjoy the classic flavors of Caesar salad with vegan Caesar dressing, a plant-based twist on a beloved classic. It's a satisfying and flavorful salad that can be enjoyed as a refreshing appetizer, side dish, or main course.

Conclusion:

Chapter 4 invites you to celebrate the vibrant and savory world of Savory Salads. These recipes demonstrate that salads can be hearty, flavorful, and a satisfying meal choice for vegans and omnivores alike. Whether you're looking for a light lunch, a refreshing side, or a substantial main course, these salads are a testament to the creativity and deliciousness of plant-based eating. So, prepare your chopping board and embrace the beauty of Savory Salads that are as nourishing as they are delightful.

Veggie Delights

Chapter 5:

Pasta Perfection.

Pasta is a universal comfort food, loved by many around the world. In this chapter 5, we dive into the world of Pasta Perfection, showcasing a collection of sumptuous and entirely plant-based pasta dishes that will satisfy your cravings for rich and comforting flavors.

1. **Creamy Cashew Alfredo:**

Start your pasta journey with a classic – Alfredo sauce. This vegan version replaces dairy with creamy cashew sauce and nutritional yeast, creating a luscious and velvety coating for your favorite pasta. Toss it with fettuccine or linguine, and you have a timeless Italian delight.

How to Prepare:

Ingredients:

For the Alfredo Sauce:

    i.   1 cup raw cashews, soaked in hot water for 1 hour

    ii.   1 cup unsweetened almond milk (or any preferred plant-based milk)

    iii.   3 cloves garlic, minced

    iv.   2 tablespoons nutritional yeast

    v.   Lemon juice- 1 teaspoon

vi.   Salt and pepper to taste

For the Pasta:

i.   12 oz fettuccine pasta (use gluten-free pasta if desired)

ii.   Fresh parsley, chopped, for garnish (optional)

Instructions:

For the Alfredo Sauce:

i.   Drain and rinse the soaked cashews.

ii.   Combine the lemon juice, soaked cashews, salt, nutritional yeast, almond milk, minced garlic, and pepper in a blender.

iii.   Blend until the mixture is smooth and creamy. You may need to scrape down the sides of the blender to ensure all ingredients are well incorporated.

For the Pasta:

i.   Cook the fettuccine pasta according to the package instructions until al dente.

ii.   Drain the pasta and return it to the pot.

iii.   Pour the creamy Alfredo sauce over the cooked pasta and toss until well coated.

iv.   Heat over low heat for a few minutes to warm the sauce.

v. Serve the creamy vegan Alfredo pasta garnished with chopped fresh parsley if desired.

Benefits:

i. **Heart-Healthy Fats:** Cashews provide healthy monounsaturated fats, which are beneficial for heart health.

ii. **Protein and Fiber:** Nutritional yeast adds protein and fiber to the sauce, promoting feelings of fullness.

iii. **Low in Saturated Fat:** This vegan Alfredo sauce is low in saturated fat and cholesterol compared to traditional dairy-based Alfredo sauce.

2. Roasted Red Pepper Pesto Linguine:

Explore the depths of flavor with a vibrant roasted red pepper pesto. Roasted red peppers, garlic, pine nuts, and fresh basil come together to create a fragrant and zesty sauce that clings perfectly to linguine. It's a pasta dish that's both visually stunning and explosively flavorful.

How to Prepare:

Ingredients:

i. 12 ounces (about 340 grams) linguine pasta (or your choice of pasta)

ii. 2 large red bell peppers

iii. 1/2 cup fresh basil leaves, packed

iv. 1/4 cup grated Parmesan cheese (or nutritional yeast for a vegan version)

v. 1/4 cup toasted pine nuts (or toasted walnuts)

vi. 2 cloves garlic, minced

vii. 1/4 cup extra-virgin olive oil

viii. Salt and black pepper to taste

ix. **Optional** garnishes: additional grated Parmesan cheese, fresh basil leaves, or red pepper flakes

Instructions:

For Roasting the Red Bell Peppers:

i. Heat the broiler or oven to high heat.

ii. Place the red bell peppers on a baking sheet or directly on the grill grates.

iii. Roast the peppers, turning occasionally, until the skin is charred and blistered on all sides. This should take about 15-20 minutes.

Remove the roasted peppers from the oven or grill and immediately transfer them to a bowl. Use a plastic wrap to cover the bowl or use a clean kitchen towel. Steam the peppers for about 10 minutes in order to be able to peel the skin more easily.

iv.

v. After steaming, peel off the charred skin from the peppers and remove the seeds and stems.

vi. Chop the roasted red peppers into smaller pieces and set aside.

For the Pesto Sauce:

i. In a food processor, combine the chopped roasted red peppers, fresh basil leaves, grated Parmesan cheese (or nutritional yeast), toasted pine nuts (or walnuts), minced garlic, and a pinch of salt and black pepper.

ii. While the food processor is running, drizzle in the extra-virgin olive oil in a steady stream until the mixture becomes smooth and well combined. You may need to scrape down the sides of the bowl with a spatula as needed.

iii. Taste the pesto and adjust the seasoning with more salt and black pepper if desired. You can also add a pinch of red pepper flakes for a hint of heat, if you like.

For Cooking the Linguine:

i. Cook the linguine pasta according to the package instructions until it's al dente. Drain and set aside.

Assembling the Roasted Red Pepper Pesto Linguine:

i. In a large serving bowl, toss the cooked linguine with the roasted red pepper pesto sauce until the pasta is well coated.

ii. If desired, garnish with additional grated Parmesan cheese, fresh basil leaves, or red pepper flakes.

iii. Serve the roasted red pepper pesto linguine hot, and enjoy!

Benefits of Roasted Red Pepper Pesto Linguine:

i. **Rich in Vitamins:** Red bell peppers are a great source of vitamin C, which supports the immune system, and vitamin A, which is important for eye health.

ii. **Healthy Fats:** Olive oil and pine nuts (or walnuts) in the pesto provide heart-healthy monounsaturated fats and omega-3 fatty acids.

iii. **Protein:** Parmesan cheese adds protein to the dish, making it more satisfying.

iv. **Antioxidants:** The combination of red bell peppers and basil in the pesto offers a variety of antioxidants that help protect cells from oxidative damage.

v. **Versatile:** This dish can be customized with additional ingredients like grilled chicken, shrimp, or roasted vegetables for added protein or variety.

vi. **Vegan Option:** You can make this dish vegan by using nutritional yeast instead of Parmesan cheese.

vii. **Flavorful:** The roasted red pepper pesto adds a rich, smoky, and slightly sweet flavor to the linguine.

viii. **Quick and Easy:** This recipe is relatively quick and easy to prepare, making it a convenient option for weeknight dinners.

Enjoy the delicious flavors and health benefits of roasted red pepper pesto linguine, a delightful combination of smoky roasted peppers, fresh basil, and toasted nuts. It's a satisfying and flavorful pasta dish that can be customized to suit your taste and dietary preferences.

3. **Spicy Arrabbiata Penne**:

If you're in the mood for some heat, look no further than the arrabbiata sauce. This spicy tomato-based sauce, infused with garlic and red pepper flakes, packs a punch. Toss it with penne pasta, and you'll have a bold and satisfying dish that's sure to awaken your taste buds.

How to Prepare:

Ingredients:

i. 12 ounces (about 340 grams) penne pasta (or your choice of pasta)
ii. 2 tablespoons olive oil
iii. 1 small onion, finely chopped
iv. 3 cloves garlic, minced
v. 1 can (14 ounces) crushed tomatoes
vi. 1/2 teaspoon red pepper flakes (adjust to taste for desired spiciness)
vii. 1 teaspoon dried oregano
viii. 1/2 teaspoon dried basil
ix. Salt and black pepper to taste
x. Fresh basil leaves for garnish (optional)
xi. Grated Parmesan cheese or nutritional yeast for serving (optional)

Instructions:

For the Sauce:

i. In a large skillet or saucepan, heat the olive oil over medium heat.
ii. Add the finely chopped onion and cook for about 2-3 minutes, or until it becomes translucent.
iii. Stir in the minced garlic and cook for another 30 seconds, or until fragrant.
iv. Add the crushed tomatoes, red pepper flakes, dried oregano, dried basil, salt, and black pepper to the skillet. Stir to combine.

v. Reduce the heat to low and simmer the sauce for about 15-20 minutes, stirring occasionally. This will allow the flavors to meld together and the sauce to thicken.

For the Penne:

i. While the sauce is simmering, cook the penne pasta in a large pot of salted boiling water according to the package instructions until it's al dente.

ii. After cooking the pasta, drain it and set it aside.

Assembling the Spicy Arrabbiata Penne:

i. Add the cooked and drained penne pasta to the spicy arrabbiata sauce in the skillet.

ii. Toss the pasta and sauce together until the pasta is evenly coated with the spicy sauce.

iii. Taste the penne and adjust the seasoning with more salt and pepper if needed.

iv. **Optionally,** garnish the spicy arrabbiata penne with fresh basil leaves for a burst of freshness.

v. Serve the penne hot, and if desired, offer grated Parmesan cheese or nutritional yeast for those who want to sprinkle some on top.

Benefits of Spicy Arrabbiata Penne:

i.   **Spicy Kick:** Red pepper flakes in the arrabbiata sauce provide a spicy kick that can stimulate the taste buds and add excitement to your meal.

ii.   **Rich in Antioxidants:** Tomatoes in the sauce are a good source of antioxidants, including lycopene, which may have various health benefits.

iii.   **Heart-Healthy:** Olive oil in the sauce is rich in monounsaturated fats, which are known for their heart-protective properties.

iv.   **Herbs and Spices:** The use of herbs like basil and oregano adds flavor without extra calories, and they may offer some health benefits.

v.   **Quick and Easy:** This recipe is relatively quick to prepare and makes for a convenient weeknight dinner option.

vi.   **Customizable:** You can adjust the level of spiciness by varying the amount of red pepper flakes, and you can add ingredients like sautéed vegetables, grilled chicken, or shrimp for added flavor and nutrition.

vii.   **Vegetarian-Friendly:** This dish is vegetarian, and you can make it vegan by using a dairy-free cheese alternative or omitting the cheese.

viii. **Comforting:** Spicy arrabbiata penne is a comforting and satisfying dish that's perfect for those who enjoy spicy flavors.

ix. **Savory and Flavorful:** The combination of garlic, onion, herbs, and tomatoes creates a savory and flavorful sauce that pairs well with penne pasta.

Enjoy the bold and spicy flavors of spicy arrabbiata penne, a simple yet satisfying pasta dish. It's a great way to add some heat and zest to your meal, and it can be tailored to your preferred level of spiciness.

4. Mushroom and Spinach Stuffed Shells:

Elevate your pasta game with these stuffed shells. Jumbo pasta shells are filled with a savory mixture of mushrooms, spinach, tofu, and herbs, then baked in marinara sauce and topped with vegan mozzarella. It's a dish that's perfect for special occasions or a hearty family dinner.

How to Prepare:

Ingredients:

For the Stuffed Shells:

i. 16 jumbo pasta shells (cooked according to package instructions)

ii.   2 cups fresh spinach, chopped

iii.   2 cups mushrooms, finely chopped (button, cremini, or any variety you prefer)

iv.   1 cup ricotta cheese (or a dairy-free alternative)

v.   1/2 cup grated Parmesan cheese (or nutritional yeast for a vegan version)

vi.   1/2 cup shredded mozzarella cheese (or a dairy-free alternative)

vii.   2 cloves garlic, minced

viii.   1 teaspoon dried basil

ix.   Salt and black pepper to taste

For the Tomato Sauce:

i.   2 cups marinara sauce (store-bought or homemade)

ii.   1/2 teaspoon dried oregano

iii.   1/2 teaspoon dried thyme

iv.   1/2 teaspoon red pepper flakes (adjust to taste)

v.   Salt and black pepper to taste

Instructions:

For the Stuffed Shells:

i.   Cook the jumbo pasta shells according to the package instructions until they are al dente. Drain and set aside.

ii. In a large skillet, heat a tablespoon of olive oil over medium heat. Add the minced garlic and chopped mushrooms. Sauté for about 5-7 minutes, or until the mushrooms release their moisture and become tender. Season with a pinch of salt and black pepper.

iii. Add the chopped spinach to the skillet and continue to cook for another 2-3 minutes, or until the spinach wilts. Remove the skillet from heat.

iv. In a mixing bowl, combine the sautéed mushroom and spinach mixture with the ricotta cheese, grated Parmesan cheese (or nutritional yeast), shredded mozzarella cheese (or dairy-free alternative), dried basil, and additional salt and black pepper to taste.

For the Tomato Sauce:

i. In a separate saucepan, heat the marinara sauce over low heat. Add dried oregano, dried thyme, red pepper flakes, salt, and black pepper. Stir to combine and let the sauce simmer for a few minutes.

Assembling the Mushroom and Spinach Stuffed Shells:

i. Heat the oven to 190°C (375°F).

ii.   Take a spoonful layer of the tomato sauce into the bottom of the baking dish. This is to prevent sticking.

iii.   Fill each cooked jumbo pasta shell with a generous spoonful of the mushroom and spinach ricotta mixture.

iv.   Place the filled shells in the baking dish, arranging them in a single layer.

v.   Pour the remaining tomato sauce over the stuffed shells, making sure they are well covered.

vi.   If you like, you can further sprinkle mozzarella cheese or grated Parmesan cheese (or vegan alternatives) over the top.

vii.   Using aluminum foil cover the baking dish. Then bake in the now hot oven for about 20-25 minutes, or until the shells are heated through and the cheese is bubbly.

viii.   Now, remove the foil and bake for another 5-10 minutes, or when you see the top is lightly golden.

ix.   Garnish with fresh basil leaves if desired.

x.   Serve the mushroom and spinach stuffed shells hot, and enjoy!

Benefits of Mushroom and Spinach Stuffed Shells:

i. **Rich in Vegetables:** Spinach and mushrooms provide essential vitamins, minerals, and antioxidants, contributing to overall health.

ii. **Protein and Calcium:** Ricotta cheese (or dairy-free alternatives) offers protein and calcium, important for muscle and bone health.

iii. **Dietary Fiber:** Spinach and whole wheat pasta shells provide dietary fiber, supporting digestive health and helping maintain satiety.

iv. **Customizable:** You can customize the filling with your favorite ingredients, such as other vegetables, herbs, or different types of cheeses.

v. **Low in Saturated Fat:** This recipe can be prepared with reduced-fat cheese for a lower saturated fat content.

vi. **Savory and Comforting:** Stuffed shells are a comforting and flavorful dish that can satisfy your craving for a hearty meal.

vii. **Make-Ahead:** You can prepare the stuffed shells in advance and bake them when you're ready to enjoy.

viii. **Vegetarian/Vegan Options:** This recipe can easily be adapted to vegetarian or vegan diets by choosing appropriate cheese and dairy-free alternatives.

Mushroom and spinach stuffed shells offer a combination of creamy and savory flavors with the goodness of vegetables and protein. It's a satisfying and comforting dish that can be enjoyed as a main course or as part of a larger meal.

5. **Lemon Garlic Spaghetti with Asparagus:**

Enjoy the brightness of lemon and garlic in this delightful spaghetti dish. Fresh asparagus spears and cherry tomatoes add a burst of color and freshness to this pasta. It's a simple yet elegant meal that's perfect for a quick weeknight dinner.

How to Prepare:

Ingredients:

i. 8 ounces (about 225 grams) spaghetti or linguine

ii. 1 bunch fresh asparagus, trimmed and cut into 2-inch pieces

iii. 3 cloves garlic, minced

iv. Zest of 1 lemon

v. Juice of 1 lemon

vi. 2 tablespoons extra-virgin olive oil

vii. 2 tablespoons unsalted butter (or a dairy-free alternative)

viii. Add black pepper and sugar to your taste

ix. Grated Parmesan cheese or nutritional yeast for serving (optional)

x.   Fresh parsley or basil leaves for garnish (optional)

Instructions:

i.   Boil salted water in a large pot. Follow the package instructions to cook the spaghetti until it's al dente. Add the asparagus pieces to the boiling water 1-2 minutes before the pasta is done. This will blanch the asparagus and cook it slightly. Drain the pasta and asparagus together.

ii.   In a large skillet, heat the olive oil and butter over medium heat. Add the minced garlic and sauté for about 30 seconds, or until fragrant. Be careful not to let it brown.

iii.   Add the cooked pasta and asparagus to the skillet with the garlic-infused oil and butter.

iv.   Toss the pasta and asparagus together to combine. Add the lemon zest and lemon juice, and continue to toss to coat the pasta evenly.

v.   Season the dish with salt and black pepper to taste. Adjust the seasoning as needed.

vi.   **Optionally**, garnish the lemon garlic spaghetti with grated Parmesan cheese or nutritional yeast for a savory, cheesy flavor.

vii.   If desired, finish with fresh parsley or basil leaves for a burst of freshness.

viii.   Serve the lemon garlic spaghetti with asparagus hot, and enjoy!

Benefits of Lemon Garlic Spaghetti with Asparagus:

i.   **Rich in Vitamins:** Asparagus is a good source of vitamins, including vitamin K, vitamin C, and folate, which support various aspects of health.

ii.   **Fiber:** Whole wheat pasta and asparagus provide dietary fiber, aiding digestion and promoting a feeling of fullness.

iii.   **Healthy Fats:** Olive oil and butter (or a dairy-free alternative) offer monounsaturated and polyunsaturated fats that support heart health.

iv.   **Antioxidants:** Lemon zest and juice provide antioxidants, including vitamin C, which can help protect your cells from oxidative stress.

v.   **Low in Saturated Fat:** This dish can be prepared with reduced-fat butter or dairy-free alternatives for a lower saturated fat content.

vi.   **Customizable:** You can customize this dish by adding ingredients like roasted cherry tomatoes, grilled chicken, or shrimp for added flavor and protein.

vii. **Vegan-Friendly:** You can make this dish vegan by using a dairy-free butter substitute and omitting the Parmesan cheese.

viii. **Quick and Easy:** Lemon garlic spaghetti with asparagus is a quick and easy recipe that's perfect for busy weeknights.

ix. **Light and Fresh:** The lemon and garlic flavors add a refreshing and zesty twist to the dish, making it a delightful spring or summer meal.

x. **Versatile:** This dish can be served as a light main course or as a side dish to complement grilled meats or seafood.

Enjoy the bright and zesty flavors of lemon garlic spaghetti with asparagus, a light and refreshing pasta dish that's perfect for a quick and delicious meal. It combines the goodness of asparagus with the tangy kick of lemon and garlic, creating a delightful balance of flavors.

6. Spicy Tomato Basil Pasta:

How to Prepare:

Ingredients:

Veggie Delights

i.   12 oz spaghetti (use gluten-free spaghetti if desired)
ii.   2 tablespoons olive oil
iii.   3 cloves garlic, minced
iv.   1/2 teaspoon red pepper flakes (adjust to your desired level of spiciness)
v.   1 can of crushed tomatoes- (28 oz)
vi.   1/2 cup fresh basil leaves, chopped
vii.   Salt and pepper to taste
viii.   Vegan Parmesan cheese for garnish (optional)

Instructions:

i.   Cook the spaghetti according to the package instructions until al dente.
ii.   In a large skillet, heat the olive oil over medium heat.
iii.   Add the minced garlic and red pepper flakes and sauté for about 1 minute until fragrant.
iv.   Pour in the crushed tomatoes and chopped basil. Stir to combine.
v.   Simmer the sauce for about 10 minutes, allowing the flavors to meld. Season with salt and pepper to taste.
vi.   Drain the cooked spaghetti and add it to the skillet with the spicy tomato basil sauce. Toss to coat the pasta evenly.

vii.   Serve the spicy tomato basil pasta hot, garnished with vegan Parmesan cheese if desired.

Benefits:

i.   **Lycopene-Rich:** Tomatoes are a great source of lycopene, an antioxidant known for its potential to reduce the risk of chronic diseases.

ii.   **Herbal Goodness:** Fresh basil not only adds flavor but also contributes to the dish's antioxidant content.

iii.   **Low in Saturated Fat:** This vegan pasta dish is low in saturated fat and cholesterol compared to dishes made with animal products. Tips and Tricks: Throughout the chapter, you'll find invaluable tips and tricks to perfect your pasta dishes. Learn how to cook pasta to the ideal al dente texture, create balanced and flavorful sauces, and pair pasta shapes with the right sauces for a satisfying and authentic experience.

Conclusion:

Chapter 5 is an invitation to indulge in the comforting embrace of Pasta Perfection. These recipes showcase the versatility and richness of vegan pasta dishes, proving that you don't need dairy or meat to enjoy a satisfying plate of pasta. Whether you're in the mood for creamy, zesty, or spicy, these pasta creations will satisfy your cravings and warm your heart. So, boil the water, cook up your favorite pasta, and savor the delicious world of plant-based pasta perfection.

Chapter 6:

Hearty Vegan Mains.

Chapter 6 presents a collection of hearty vegan main course dishes that are not only delicious but also packed with health benefits. These recipes showcase the versatility of plant-based ingredients in creating satisfying and nourishing meals. Below, you'll find instructions on how to prepare two standout dishes from this chapter along with their associated benefits:

1. Spicy Chickpea Curry:

How to Prepare:

Ingredients:

i. 2 tablespoons coconut oil

ii. 1 large onion, finely chopped

iii. 3 cloves garlic, minced

iv. An inch piece of minced fresh ginger

v. 1 tablespoon curry powder

vi. 1 teaspoon ground cumin

vii. 1 teaspoon ground coriander

viii. 1/2 teaspoon ground turmeric

ix. 1/4 teaspoon cayenne pepper (adjust to your spice preference)

x. 1 (14 oz) can of diced tomatoes

xi. 2 (14 oz) cans of chickpeas, drained and rinsed

xii. 1 (14 oz) can of coconut milk

xiii. Salt and pepper to taste

xiv. Fresh cilantro, chopped, for garnish (optional)

Instructions:

i. In a large skillet, heat the coconut oil over medium heat.

ii. Add the chopped onion and sauté until translucent, about 5 minutes.

iii. Stir in the minced garlic, ginger, curry powder, cumin, coriander, turmeric, and cayenne pepper. Cook for another 2 minutes until fragrant.

iv. Add the diced tomatoes, chickpeas, and coconut milk. Stir to combine.

v. Simmer the curry over low heat for 15-20 minutes, allowing the flavors to meld and the sauce to thicken.

vi. Season with salt and pepper to taste.

vii. Garnish with fresh chopped cilantro before serving, if desired.

viii. Serve the spicy chickpea curry with rice or naan bread.

Benefits:

i. **Plant-Based Protein:** Chickpeas are a rich source of plant-based protein, aiding in muscle repair and overall health.

ii. **Antioxidants:** The spices in this curry, such as turmeric and cumin, contain antioxidants that may help reduce inflammation.

iii. **Coconut Milk:** Coconut milk provides healthy fats and a creamy texture, making the curry satisfying and nutritious.

2. Vegan BBQ Pulled Jackfruit Sandwiches

Ingredients:

For the BBQ Sauce:

i. Tomato sauce- (1 cup)
ii. 1/4 cup tomato paste
iii. 1/4 cup apple cider vinegar
iv. 2 tablespoons maple syrup
v. 1 tablespoon smoked paprika
vi. 1 teaspoon garlic powder
vii. 1 teaspoon onion powder
viii. Salt and pepper to taste

For the Pulled Jackfruit:

i. 2 (20 oz) cans of young green jackfruit in water or brine, drained and rinsed
ii. 1 onion, finely chopped
iii. Minced garlic- (2 cloves)
iv. 1 tablespoon olive oil
v. 1/4 cup vegetable broth
vi. Salt and pepper to taste

vii.   4 whole wheat or gluten-free buns

Instructions:

For the BBQ Sauce:

i.   In a saucepan, combine all the BBQ sauce ingredients and whisk together.

ii.   Simmer over low heat for about 10 minutes, stirring occasionally. Adjust seasonings to taste.

For the Pulled Jackfruit:

i.   In a large skillet, heat the olive oil over medium heat.

ii.   Add the chopped onion and sauté until translucent, about 5 minutes.

iii.   Stir in the minced garlic and cook for another minute.

iv.   Add the drained jackfruit and vegetable broth. Use a fork or potato masher to break apart the jackfruit into shreds.

v.   Pour in the prepared BBQ sauce and stir to coat the jackfruit thoroughly.

vi.   Simmer for 10-15 minutes over low heat, allowing the flavors to meld and the jackfruit to absorb the sauce.

vii.   Season with salt and pepper to taste.

viii.   Serve the pulled jackfruit BBQ on whole wheat or gluten-free buns.

Benefits:

i. **Jackfruit Nutritional Value:** Jackfruit is a good source of dietary fiber, vitamin C, and various B vitamins, making it a nutritious meat substitute.

ii. **Low in Fat:** This vegan BBQ pulled jackfruit is naturally low in fat and cholesterol, supporting heart health.

iii. **Whole Wheat Buns:** Whole wheat buns provide complex carbohydrates and dietary fiber for sustained energy.

These hearty vegan mains from Chapter 6 offered you a delicious way to enjoy plant-based meals that are both satisfying and nutritious. Whether you opt for the bold and spicy Chickpea Curry or the savory and smoky Vegan BBQ Pulled Jackfruit Sandwiches, these dishes showcase the potential of vegan cooking to create flavorful and wholesome main courses.

Veggie Delights

Chapter 7:

Side Dish Delights.

Side dishes may play a supporting role at the dinner table, but in this chapter, we celebrate these unsung heroes that can transform a meal into a culinary masterpiece. These Side Dish Delights are not just accompaniments but stars in their own right, offering a world of flavors, textures, and colors to complement your main courses.

1. **Garlic Roasted Brussels Sprouts:**

Elevate Brussels sprouts from the often-dismissed vegetable tray to the realm of delectable side dishes. Oven-roasting with garlic, olive oil, and a sprinkle of sea salt brings out their natural sweetness and a delightful crunch. These garlic roasted Brussels sprouts are perfect for adding a savory, nutty dimension to any meal.

How to Prepare:

Ingredients:

    i.   1 pound Brussels sprouts
    ii.   3-4 cloves garlic, minced
    iii.   2-3 tablespoons olive oil
    iv.   Salt and pepper to taste
    v.   **Optional:** grated Parmesan cheese or balsamic vinegar for added flavor

Instructions:

i. **Preheat the Oven:** Preheat your oven to 400°F (200°C).

ii. **Prepare the Brussels Sprouts:** Trim the stem ends of the Brussels sprouts and remove any loose or damaged leaves. Cut each Brussels sprout in half lengthwise.

iii. **Season:** In a large bowl, combine the halved Brussels sprouts, minced garlic, olive oil, salt, and pepper. Toss everything together until the Brussels sprouts are well-coated with the garlic and oil mixture.

iv. **Roast:** Spread the seasoned Brussels sprouts evenly on a baking sheet or in a baking dish, making sure they are in a single layer for even cooking. Place them in the preheated oven.

v. **Roast:** Roast the Brussels sprouts for about 20-25 minutes or until they are tender and have developed a nice golden brown color. You can toss them halfway through the cooking time for even browning.

vi. **Serve:** Once roasted, remove the Brussels sprouts from the oven. If desired, sprinkle some grated Parmesan cheese or drizzle balsamic vinegar over them for extra flavor before serving.

Benefits of Garlic Roasted Brussels Sprouts:

i. **Rich in Nutrients:** Brussels sprouts are an excellent source of vitamins C and K, as well as folate, vitamin B6, and various minerals like potassium and manganese.

ii. **High in Fiber:** They are a good source of dietary fiber, which can aid in digestion and help you feel full and satisfied.

iii. **Antioxidant Properties:** Brussels sprouts contain antioxidants like vitamin C and vitamin A, which can help protect your cells from damage caused by free radicals.

iv. **Heart Health:** The fiber and potassium in Brussels sprouts can contribute to heart health by helping to lower blood pressure and reduce the risk of cardiovascular disease.

v. **Cancer Prevention:** Some studies suggest that compounds in Brussels sprouts may have cancer-fighting properties, particularly against certain types of cancers.

vi. **Low in Calories:** Brussels sprouts are relatively low in calories, making them a healthy addition to your diet, especially if you're watching your calorie intake.

vii. **Delicious Flavor:** Roasting Brussels sprouts with garlic and olive oil enhances their natural flavor, making them a tasty and enjoyable side dish.

Garlic Roasted Brussels Sprouts can be a versatile addition to your meals, whether you serve them as a side dish, add them to salads, or use them in various recipes. Enjoy the health benefits and delicious taste of this nutritious vegetable dish.

2. Buttered Mashed Sweet Potatoes:

Experience the comforting embrace of creamy mashed sweet potatoes, a vegan twist on a classic favorite. With a hint of cinnamon, nutmeg, and a dollop of vegan butter, these mashed sweet potatoes are both satisfying and indulgent. They pair beautifully with roasted vegetables, vegan roasts, or as a standalone side dish.

How to prepare:

Ingredients:

i. 3-4 medium sweet potatoes
ii. 2-3 tablespoons butter
iii. Salt and pepper to taste
iv. **Optional:** a pinch of cinnamon or nutmeg for added flavor

v. **Optional toppings:** chopped fresh herbs, toasted pecans, or marshmallows for garnish

Instructions:

i. **Prepare the Sweet Potatoes:** Wash and peel the sweet potatoes. Cut them into chunks or slices for quicker cooking.

ii. **Boil the Sweet Potatoes:** Place the sweet potato chunks in a large pot and cover them with water. Put a small quantity of salt to the water. Let the water boil, then cook the sweet potatoes. Let it cook until they are soft. This takes about 15-20 minutes.

iii. **Drain and Mash:** Drain the cooked sweet potatoes in a colander. Return them to the pot and use a potato masher or a fork to mash them to your desired consistency. You can make them as smooth or as chunky as you like.

iv. **Add Butter and Seasonings:** Add the butter to the mashed sweet potatoes while they are still hot. The heat from the sweet potatoes will melt the butter. Stir the butter into the sweet potatoes until it's well incorporated. Season with salt, pepper, and any optional spices like cinnamon or nutmeg. Adjust the seasonings to taste.

v. **Serve:** Transfer the buttered mashed sweet potatoes to a serving dish. If desired, garnish with chopped fresh herbs, toasted pecans, or marshmallows before serving.

Benefits of Buttered Mashed Sweet Potatoes:

i. **Rich in Nutrients:** Sweet potatoes are an excellent source of vitamins and minerals, including vitamin A (in the form of beta-carotene), vitamin C, potassium, and fiber.

ii. **Antioxidant Properties:** The orange flesh of sweet potatoes contains antioxidants that help protect your cells from damage caused by free radicals.

iii. **Good for Eye Health:** The beta-carotene in sweet potatoes is essential for good vision and may help prevent age-related eye diseases.

iv. **Digestive Health:** The fiber in sweet potatoes can aid in digestion and promote a healthy gut.

v. **Immune Support:** Vitamin C in sweet potatoes plays a role in supporting your immune system and overall health.

vi. **Satisfying and Comforting:** Mashed sweet potatoes have a naturally sweet flavor that is both satisfying and comforting, making them a great addition to any meal.

vii. **Versatile:** You can customize the flavor of mashed sweet potatoes with various seasonings and toppings, making them a versatile side dish for different occasions.

Buttered Mashed Sweet Potatoes are not only nutritious but also a crowd-pleaser due to their sweet and creamy texture. Whether you serve them alongside a holiday roast or as a comforting side dish for everyday meals, they are sure to be a hit.

3. **Herbed Quinoa Pilaf:**

Quinoa takes center stage in this flavorful side dish. Cooked with aromatic herbs, sautéed onions, and vegetable broth, this quinoa pilaf is a delightful blend of savory and nutty flavors. It's the perfect accompaniment to grilled tofu, roasted vegetables, or as a stuffing for bell peppers.

How to Prepare:

Ingredients:

i.   1 cup quinoa
ii.   2 cups vegetable broth or water
iii.   Butter or olive oil- 2 tablespoons
iv.   A finely chopped onion
v.   2 cloves garlic, minced
vi.   1 carrot, diced

vii.   1 celery stalk, diced

viii.   1 red bell pepper, diced

ix.   1/2 cup frozen peas (or fresh if available)

x.   1/4 cup fresh herbs (such as parsley, basil, and chives), chopped

xi.   Salt and pepper to taste

xii.   **Optional:** 1/4 cup toasted nuts (such as almonds or pine nuts) for garnish

Instructions:

i.   **Rinse the Quinoa:** Rinse the quinoa thoroughly under cold running water to remove any bitterness. Drain well.

ii.   **Toast the Quinoa:** In a large saucepan or skillet, heat the olive oil or butter over medium heat. Add the quinoa and toast it for about 2-3 minutes, stirring frequently, until it starts to smell nutty and turn a slightly golden color.

iii.   **Add Aromatics:** Add the chopped onion and garlic to the toasted quinoa. Sauté for 2-3 minutes until the onion becomes translucent and fragrant.

iv.   **Add Vegetables:** Stir in the diced carrot, celery, and red bell pepper. Fry while continuously stirring for another 3-4 minutes until the vegetables softens.

v.   **Cook Quinoa:** Pour in the vegetable broth or water and bring the mixture to a boil. Reduce the heat to low, cover the saucepan, and let it simmer for about 15-20 minutes, or until the liquid is absorbed and the quinoa is tender.

vi. **Fluff and Add Peas:** Once the quinoa is cooked, fluff it with a fork and stir in the frozen peas. Cover and let it sit for a few minutes until the peas are heated through.

vii. **Herbs and Seasoning:** Remove the quinoa pilaf from heat. Stir in the freshly chopped herbs (parsley, basil, and chives work well). Season with salt and pepper to taste.

viii. **Garnish and Serve:** If desired, garnish the herbed quinoa pilaf with toasted nuts (e.g., almonds or pine nuts) for added flavor and texture. Serve hot as a side dish or as a light, nutritious meal.

Benefits of Herbed Quinoa Pilaf:

i. **High-Quality Protein:** Quinoa is a complete protein source, containing all nine essential amino acids, making it an excellent choice for vegetarians and vegans.

ii. **Rich in Fiber:** Quinoa is a good source of dietary fiber, which aids in digestion and helps maintain a feeling of fullness.

iii. **Nutrient-Rich:** Quinoa is rich in vitamins and minerals, including manganese, phosphorus, magnesium, and folate.

iv. **Low Glycemic Index:** Quinoa has a low glycemic index, which means it can help regulate blood sugar levels.

v. **Antioxidant Properties:** The herbs and vegetables in this dish provide antioxidants that help protect cells from damage caused by free radicals.

vi. **Heart-Healthy:** Quinoa is known to support heart health due to its high fiber and potassium content.

vii. **Versatile:** You can customize the herbed quinoa pilaf with various herbs and vegetables to suit your taste preferences and what's in season.

Herbed Quinoa Pilaf is not only nutritious but also versatile and delicious. It can be served as a side dish or as a light and healthy main course. Enjoy the fresh, herbaceous flavors and the numerous health benefits of this dish.

4. Lemon Garlic Roasted Asparagus:

Transform fresh asparagus into a zesty and aromatic delight. Roasted with lemon zest, minced garlic, and a drizzle of olive oil, this side dish is a burst of freshness and flavor. Serve it alongside pasta dishes, vegan protein, or as an elegant addition to your holiday table.

How to Prepare:

Ingredients:

i.   1 bunch of fresh asparagus spears

ii.   2-3 cloves garlic, minced

iii.   Zest of 1 lemon

iv.   Juice of half a lemon

v.   2-3 tablespoons olive oil

vi.   Salt and freshly ground black pepper, to taste

vii. **Optional:** grated Parmesan cheese or toasted almonds for garnish

Instructions:

i.   **Preheat the Oven:** Preheat your oven to 400°F (200°C).

ii.   **Prepare the Asparagus:** Wash the asparagus spears and trim the tough, woody ends. You can do this by holding one end of the spear and bending it; it will naturally snap where the tough part ends. Discard the tough ends.

iii. **Season the Asparagus:** In a large bowl, toss the trimmed asparagus spears with minced garlic, lemon zest, lemon juice, olive oil, salt, and freshly ground black pepper. Make sure the asparagus is evenly coated with the mixture.

iv. **Roast the Asparagus:** Place the seasoned asparagus in a single layer on a baking sheet or in a baking dish. Roast in the preheated oven for about 12-15 minutes, or until the asparagus is tender and slightly crispy at the tips. The cooking time may vary depending on the thickness of the asparagus spears.

v. **Garnish and Serve:** Remove the roasted asparagus from the oven and, if desired, sprinkle with grated Parmesan cheese or toasted almonds for added flavor and texture. Serve immediately.

Benefits of Lemon Garlic Roasted Asparagus:

i. **High in Fiber:** Asparagus is a good source of dietary fiber, which aids in digestion and helps maintain a feeling of fullness.

ii. **Rich in Vitamins:** Asparagus is particularly high in vitamins like vitamin K, vitamin A, vitamin C, and several B vitamins, including folate.

iii. **Mineral-Rich:** It contains essential minerals such as potassium, phosphorus, and calcium.

iv. **Antioxidant Properties:** Asparagus is rich in antioxidants like vitamins A and C, which help protect your cells from damage caused by free radicals.

v. **Low in Calories:** Asparagus is low in calories and can be a great addition to a balanced diet, especially if you're watching your calorie intake.

vi. **Diuretic Properties:** Asparagus contains asparagine, a natural diuretic, which may help with reducing water retention.

vii. **Delicious Flavor:** Roasting asparagus with garlic and lemon enhances its natural flavors, making it a tasty and satisfying side dish.

Lemon Garlic Roasted Asparagus is a versatile side dish that pairs well with various main courses, and it's a great way to enjoy the benefits of this nutritious vegetable. It's not only delicious but also quick and easy to prepare, making it a perfect addition to your meals.

5. Balsamic Glazed Carrots:

Elevate humble carrots with a balsamic glaze. Roasted until tender and then drizzled with a sweet and tangy balsamic reduction, these carrots become a standout side dish that pairs beautifully with roasted potatoes, vegan steaks, or a simple grain-based salad.

How to Prepare:

Ingredients:

i.   1 pound (about 4 cups) carrots, peeled and sliced into 1/4-inch thick rounds or diagonal coins

ii.   2 tablespoons olive oil

iii.   2-3 tablespoons balsamic vinegar

iv.   2 tablespoons honey or maple syrup (for sweetness)

v.   2 cloves garlic, minced

vi.   Salt and freshly ground black pepper to taste

vii.   (Optional) Chives for garnish or Fresh parsley

Instructions:

i.   **Prepare the Carrots:** Peel and slice the carrots into rounds or diagonal coins, ensuring they are of uniform thickness for even cooking.

ii.   **Cook the Carrots:** In a large skillet, heat the olive oil over medium-high heat. Add the sliced carrots and sauté for about 5 minutes, or until they start to develop some color and become slightly tender.

iii. **Add Flavor:** Stir in the minced garlic and sauté for another 30 seconds to 1 minute until fragrant.

iv. **Glaze the Carrots:** Pour in the balsamic vinegar and honey or maple syrup. Stir well to coat the carrots evenly. Reduce the heat to medium-low and let the carrots simmer for 5-7 minutes, or until the balsamic mixture thickens and glazes the carrots. Stir occasionally to prevent burning.

v. **Season and Garnish:** Season the glazed carrots with salt and freshly ground black pepper to taste. If desired, garnish with fresh parsley or chives for a burst of color and added flavor.

vi. **Serve:** Transfer the balsamic glazed carrots to a serving dish and serve hot.

Benefits of Balsamic Glazed Carrots:

i. **Rich in Nutrients:** Carrots are packed with vitamins and minerals, particularly vitamin A, vitamin K, vitamin C, and potassium.

ii. **Dietary Fiber:** Carrots are a good source of dietary fiber, which supports digestion and helps maintain a feeling of fullness.

iii. **Antioxidants:** Carrots contain antioxidants, such as beta-carotene, which can help protect your cells from oxidative stress and reduce the risk of chronic diseases.

iv. **Blood Sugar Regulation:** The fiber and natural sugars in carrots may help regulate blood sugar levels.

v. **Heart Health:** Carrots are low in saturated fats and cholesterol and can be part of a heart-healthy diet.

vi. **Tasty and Versatile:** Balsamic glaze adds a rich and tangy flavor to the carrots, making them a delicious side dish that complements a wide range of main courses.

Balsamic Glazed Carrots are a delightful way to enjoy the natural sweetness of carrots with a touch of acidity from the balsamic vinegar. They are a colorful and nutritious addition to your meal, and the glaze enhances their flavor profile. This dish is sure to be a hit with both kids and adults alike.

Chapter 8:

Decadent Desserts.

Desserts are the grand finale of any meal, and in Chapter 8 of "Veggie Delights," we venture into the realm of Decadent Desserts. These plant-based sweet treats prove that vegan desserts are not only delicious but also indulgent, satisfying your sweet tooth while aligning with your ethical choices. From creamy delights to fruity sensations, this chapter offers a delightful array of vegan desserts to satisfy your cravings.

1. Chocolate Avocado Mousse:

Experience the magic of avocados in dessert form with a rich and velvety chocolate avocado mousse. Ripe avocados blend seamlessly with cocoa powder, maple syrup, and a hint of vanilla to create a creamy and satisfying treat. This dessert comes out as the fulfillment of the chocolate-lover's dream

How to Prepare:

Ingredients:

i.	2 ripe avocados, peeled and pitted
ii.	1/4 cup unsweetened cocoa powder
iii.	1/4 cup maple syrup or agave nectar
iv.	1 teaspoon vanilla extract
v.	A pinch of salt
vi.	Fresh berries for garnish (optional)

Instructions:

i. Place the peeled and pitted avocados in a food processor or blender.

ii. Add the cocoa powder, maple syrup or agave nectar, vanilla extract, and a pinch of salt.

iii. Blend until the mixture is smooth and creamy, scraping down the sides as needed.

iv. Spoon the chocolate avocado mousse into serving dishes.

v. Chill in the refrigerator for at least 30 minutes to firm up.

vi. Garnish with fresh berries before serving, if desired.

Benefits:

i. **Healthy Fats:** Avocado provides healthy monounsaturated fats that are good for heart health.

ii. **Antioxidants:** Cocoa powder is rich in antioxidants called flavonoids, which may have various health benefits.

iii. **Natural Sweetener:** Maple syrup or agave nectar adds sweetness without refined sugars.

2. **Creamy Coconut Rice Pudding:**

Delve into the comforting embrace of creamy coconut rice pudding. Arborio rice simmers in coconut milk until tender, absorbing the sweet and tropical flavors. Infused with a touch of vanilla and garnished with toasted coconut flakes, this dessert is a warm and delightful treat.

How to Prepare:

Ingredients:

i.   1 cup white rice (short-grain or jasmine rice works well)

ii.   1 can (13.5 ounces) coconut milk (full-fat for creaminess)

iii.   1/2 cup sugar (adjust to taste)

iv.   1/2 teaspoon vanilla extract

v.   Salt- (1/4 teaspoon)

vi.   1/4 teaspoon ground cinnamon (optional)

vii.   1/4 cup shredded coconut (optional, for garnish)

viii.   Fresh fruit, such as mango or pineapple (optional, for garnish)

Instructions:

i.   **Rinse and Cook the Rice:** Rinse the rice under cold water until the water runs clear. Put the rinsed rice together in a saucepan (medium-size), with 2 cups of water. Boil the combination over a heat-(medium-high heat), then turn the heat to low. Then cover it and simmer for about 18-20 minutes. Boil until the rice is tender and the liquid is completely absorbed.

ii. **Combine Ingredients:** Once the rice is cooked, stir in the coconut milk, sugar, vanilla extract, salt, and ground cinnamon (if using). Mix everything together.

iii. **Simmer:** Place the saucepan back on the stove over low heat. Continue to cook, stirring frequently, for about 15-20 minutes until the mixture thickens and becomes creamy. Adjust the sugar taste if needed.

iv. **Cool and Serve:** Remove the coconut rice pudding from the heat. Cool it for some minutes and watch how it continues to become thicker as it gets cooler. You can serve it while chilled or warm as you prefer.

v. **Garnish:** If desired, garnish with shredded coconut and fresh fruit, such as mango or pineapple, for added flavor and presentation.

Benefits of Creamy Coconut Rice Pudding:

i. **Rich in Calories:** Coconut rice pudding is a calorie-dense dessert, making it a great source of energy when needed.

ii. **Coconut Nutrients:** Coconut milk provides healthy fats and is a good source of essential minerals like manganese, copper, and iron.

iii. **Dairy-Free:** This dessert is dairy-free, making it suitable for individuals with lactose intolerance or dairy allergies.

iv. **Gluten-Free:** Rice is naturally gluten-free, making this dessert safe for those with gluten sensitivities or celiac disease.

v. **Comforting and Satisfying:** Coconut rice pudding is a comforting and satisfying dessert, making it a great treat for special occasions or when you're craving something sweet.

vi. **Customizable:** You can customize this dessert by adjusting the level of sweetness, adding spices like cinnamon or cardamom, or garnishing with your favorite fruits and nuts.

Creamy Coconut Rice Pudding is a delightful way to enjoy the tropical flavor of coconut in a sweet and creamy dessert. It's versatile and can be enjoyed warm or chilled, making it a versatile addition to your dessert repertoire.

3. **Vegan Cheesecake with Berry Compote:**

Indulge in the elegance of a vegan cheesecake with a luscious berry compote. The creamy filling, often made with cashews or silken tofu, is perfectly sweetened and infused with vanilla. The berry compote adds a burst of fruity brightness that beautifully contrasts with the rich filling. It's a dessert that's as visually stunning as it is delicious.

How to Prepare:

Ingredients:

For the Crust:

i.   1 1/2 cups vegan graham cracker crumbs (you can use gluten-free if needed)
ii.   1/4 cup coconut oil, melted (or vegan butter)
iii.   2 tablespoons maple syrup (or another liquid sweetener)

For the Cheesecake Filling:

i.   2 cups raw cashews, soaked in hot water for 1-2 hours, then drained
ii.   1/2 cup coconut cream (the thick part from a can of full-fat coconut milk)
iii.   1/2 cup lemon juice
iv.   1/2 cup maple syrup (adjust to taste)
v.   1/4 cup coconut oil, melted

vi.   1 teaspoon vanilla extract

vii.   A pinch of salt

For the Berry Compote:

i.   2 cups mixed berries (strawberries, blueberries, raspberries, etc.)

ii.   2 tablespoons maple syrup (adjust to taste)

iii.   1 tablespoon lemon juice

Instructions:

For the Crust:

i.   Preheat your oven to 350°F (175°C).

ii.   In a mixing bowl, combine the vegan graham cracker crumbs, melted coconut oil (or vegan butter), and maple syrup. Stir until the mixture resembles wet sand.

iii.   Press the mixture firmly into the bottom of a greased 9-inch (23 cm) springform pan, creating an even layer.

iv.   In the heated oven, bake the crust for about 10 minutes. As you are preparing the cheesecake filling, remove the crust from the oven and let it cool down.

For the Cheesecake Filling:

i.   In a high-powered blender or food processor, combine the soaked and drained cashews, coconut cream, lemon juice, maple syrup, melted coconut oil, vanilla extract, and a pinch of salt.

ii. Blend until the mixture is completely smooth and creamy. You may need to scrape down the sides of the blender or food processor to ensure everything is well mixed.

iii. Pour the cheesecake filling over the cooled crust in the springform pan.

iv. Smooth the top with a spatula to create an even surface.

v. Place the cheesecake in the refrigerator and let it chill for at least 4 hours or until it's set and firm.

For the Berry Compote:

i. In a saucepan, combine the mixed berries, maple syrup, and lemon juice.

ii. Heat the mixture over medium heat, stirring occasionally, until the berries break down and the mixture thickens, about 10-15 minutes.

iii. Remove from heat and let it cool.

Assembly:

i. Once the cheesecake is fully chilled and set, carefully remove it from the springform pan.

ii. Top the cheesecake with the cooled berry compote, spreading it evenly over the surface.

iii. Slice and serve your Vegan Cheesecake with Berry Compote.

Benefits of Vegan Cheesecake with Berry Compote:

i. **Dairy-Free:** This cheesecake is entirely dairy-free and suitable for vegans or those with lactose intolerance.

ii. **Plant-Based:** It's made from plant-based ingredients, making it a cruelty-free dessert option.

iii. **Healthy Fats:** The cashews and coconut oil provide healthy fats that can be part of a balanced diet.

iv. **Lower in Saturated Fat:** Compared to traditional cheesecake, which is high in saturated fat from dairy, this vegan version is lower in saturated fat.

v. **Customizable:** You can adapt the flavors and toppings to your liking, such as using different berries for the compote or adding chocolate chips to the filling.

Vegan Cheesecake with Berry Compote is a delightful dessert that satisfies your sweet tooth while adhering to vegan dietary preferences. It's rich, creamy, and bursting with the flavors of fresh berries. Enjoy it guilt-free as a treat or for special occasions.

4. **Classic Apple Crisp:**

Savor the nostalgia of a classic apple crisp with a vegan twist. Sliced apples, seasoned with cinnamon and sugar, are baked until tender, while the crisp topping boasts a delightful blend of oats, flour, and vegan butter. Serve it warm with a scoop of vegan vanilla ice cream for the perfect dessert.

How to Prepare:

Ingredients:

For the Apple Filling:

i. 6-8 cups of sliced and peeled apples (such as Granny Smith, Honeycrisp, or Fuji)
ii. Sugar (granulated)- half a cup
iii. 1 tablespoon lemon juice
iv. 1 teaspoon ground cinnamon
v. 1/4 teaspoon ground nutmeg (optional)
vi. 1/4 teaspoon salt

For the Crisp Topping:

i. Rolled oats (old-fashioned)- a cup
ii. 1/2 cup all-purpose flour (or a gluten-free flour blend)
iii. 1/2 cup brown sugar (packed)

    iv.   1/2 teaspoon ground cinnamon

    v.   1/4 teaspoon salt

    vi.   1/2 cup (1 stick) unsalted butter or vegan butter substitute, cold and diced

Instructions:

i. **Preheat the Oven**: Preheat your oven to 350°F (175°C).

ii. **Prepare the Apple Filling**: In a large mixing bowl, combine the sliced and peeled apples with the granulated sugar, lemon juice, ground cinnamon, ground nutmeg (if using), and salt. Toss everything together until the apples are evenly coated.

iii. **Transfer to Baking Dish**: Transfer the apple mixture to a 9x13-inch (23x33 cm) baking dish or a similar-sized ovenproof dish, spreading it out evenly.

iv. **Prepare the Crisp** Topping: In a different bowl, combine the all-purpose flour, oats, salt, brown sugar, ground cinnamon and stir to mix

v. **Add Butter:** Add the cold, diced butter (or vegan butter) to the oat mixture.

vi. **Crumble Topping**: Use a pastry cutter, two forks, or your hands to cut the butter into the oat mixture until it resembles coarse crumbs. The topping should hold together when pressed but also be crumbly.

vii. **Cover the Apples**: Sprinkle the crisp topping evenly over the apple mixture in the baking dish.

viii. **Bake**: Place the baking dish in the preheated oven and bake for 40-45 minutes or until the apple filling is bubbling, and the topping is golden brown and crispy.

ix. **Cool Slightly:** Remove the apple crisp from the oven and let it cool for a few minutes before serving. Serve at room temperature or warm.

Benefits of Classic Apple Crisp:

i. **Fiber-Rich:** Apples are a good source of dietary fiber, which supports digestive health and helps keep you feeling full.

ii. **Vitamins and Minerals:** Apples provide vitamins like vitamin C and various B vitamins, as well as minerals like potassium.

iii. **Antioxidants:** Apples contain antioxidants, particularly in their skin, that help protect your cells from oxidative damage.

iv. **Warm and Comforting:** Apple crisp is a comforting dessert, perfect for cool or chilly weather.

v. **Customizable:** You can customize your apple crisp by using different types of apples or adding ingredients like chopped nuts or raisins to the topping.

vi. **Family Favorite:** It's a dessert loved by many and often enjoyed during family gatherings and holidays.

Classic Apple Crisp is a timeless dessert that combines the natural sweetness of apples with a crunchy, buttery topping. It's a crowd-pleaser and a wonderful way to enjoy the flavors of fall or indulge in a comforting treat year-round. Serve it with a scoop of vanilla ice cream or a dollop of whipped cream for an extra special treat.

5. Banana Chocolate Chip Bread:

Embrace the comforting aroma of freshly baked banana chocolate chip bread. Ripe bananas and dairy-free chocolate chips create a moist and flavorful loaf that's perfect for breakfast, brunch, or dessert. Slice it thick and enjoy with a cup of hot tea or coffee.

How to Prepare:

Ingredients:

i. 2 to 3 ripe bananas, mashed (about 1 cup)
ii. 1/3 cup melted butter or vegetable oil
iii. 3/4 cup granulated sugar
iv. 1 large egg
v. Vanilla extract- (1 teaspoon)
vi. 1 1/2 cups all-purpose flour
vii. 1 teaspoon baking soda
viii. 1/2 teaspoon baking powder
ix. 1/2 teaspoon salt
x. 1/2 cup chocolate chips (you can use semi-sweet, milk chocolate, or dark chocolate chips)

Instructions:

i. **Preheat the Oven:** Preheat your oven to 350°F (175°C). Grease a 9x5-inch (23x13 cm) loaf pan or line it with parchment paper for easy removal.

ii. **Mash the Bananas:** In a mixing bowl, mash the ripe bananas using a fork until they are mostly smooth with a few small lumps.

iii. **Combine Wet Ingredients:** Add the melted butter or vegetable oil to the mashed bananas and stir until well combined. Then, add the granulated sugar, egg, and vanilla extract. Mix until the wet ingredients are thoroughly combined.

iv. **Sift Dry Ingredients:** In a separate bowl, sift together the all-purpose flour, baking soda, baking powder, and salt.

v. **Combine Wet and Dry Ingredients:** Gradually add the sifted dry ingredients to the banana mixture, stirring until just combined. Be careful not to overmix; it's okay if there are a few small lumps.

vi. **Add Chocolate Chips:** Gently fold in the chocolate chips until they are evenly distributed throughout the batter.

vii. **Transfer to Loaf Pan:** Pour the batter into the prepared loaf pan, spreading it out evenly.

viii. **Bake:** Bake in the preheated oven for about 60-70 minutes or until a toothpick or cake tester inserted into the center of the bread comes out clean or with a few moist crumbs attached.

ix. **Cool and Serve:** Remove the banana chocolate chip bread from the oven and allow it to cool in the pan for about 10-15 minutes. Then, transfer it to a wire rack to cool completely before slicing.

Benefits of Banana Chocolate Chip Bread:

i. **Rich in Potassium:** Bananas are a good source of potassium, which is important

<ol type="i">
<li value="1">for maintaining healthy blood pressure and proper muscle function.</li>
<li>Fiber Content: Bananas are rich in dietary fiber, which aids in digestion and helps regulate bowel movements.</li>
<li>Vitamins and Minerals: Bananas provide essential vitamins and minerals, including vitamin C, vitamin B6, and manganese.</li>
<li>Antioxidants: Dark chocolate chips contain antioxidants, which may help protect cells from damage caused by free radicals.</li>
<li>Satisfying Treat: Banana chocolate chip bread is a satisfying and comforting treat that can satisfy your sweet tooth while also providing some nutritional benefits.</li>
<li>Versatile: This bread is a versatile snack or dessert that can be enjoyed for breakfast, brunch, or as a tasty snack at any time of day.</li>
</ol>

Banana Chocolate Chip Bread is a delightful way to use up overripe bananas and enjoy a sweet, moist treat. It's a crowd-pleaser that combines the goodness of bananas with the indulgence of chocolate chips, making it a favorite among both kids and adults.

Conclusion:

This chapter 8 of "Veggie Delights" made you to indulge in the world of Decadent Desserts, proving that vegan sweets are as delightful and satisfying as their non-vegan counterparts. Whether you're craving chocolate, fruit, or a comforting classic, these dessert recipes offer a spectrum of flavors and textures to satisfy your sweet tooth. So, prepare to delight in the creativity and deliciousness of plant-based desserts that will impress your guests and make every meal feel like a celebration.

Veggie Delights

Chapter 9:

International Flavors.

Chapter 9 takes you on an exciting journey across the globe to explore a myriad of international flavors. These recipes showcase the rich, diverse, and delicious world of vegan cuisine from various countries and regions. Whether you're craving the aromatic spices of India, the comforting pasta of Italy, or the exotic dishes of the Middle East, this chapter offers a passport to tantalize your taste buds.

1. **Moroccan Chickpea Tagine:**

Begin your culinary adventure with a Moroccan Chickpea Tagine, a fragrant and hearty dish that combines chickpeas, tomatoes, and a medley of spices like cumin, coriander, and cinnamon. Slow-cooked to perfection, it's traditionally served with couscous or crusty bread for a satisfying meal.

How to Prepare:

Ingredients:

For the Tagine:

i. 2 tablespoons olive oil
ii. 1 large onion, finely chopped
iii. 3 cloves garlic, minced
iv. Minced fresh ginger- (1 tablespoon)
v. 2 teaspoons ground cumin

vi.   1 teaspoon ground coriander
vii.   1 teaspoon ground paprika
viii.   1/2 teaspoon ground cinnamon
ix.   1/4 teaspoon cayenne pepper (adjust to taste)
x.   1 can (15 ounces) chickpeas, drained and rinsed
xi.   1 can (15 ounces) diced tomatoes
xii.   2 carrots, peeled and diced
xiii.   2 potatoes, peeled and diced
xiv.   1 zucchini, diced
xv.   1 red bell pepper, diced
xvi.   1 cup vegetable broth
xvii.   Salt and pepper to taste
xviii. Fresh cilantro or parsley for garnish

For the Couscous (optional):

i.   1 cup couscous
ii.   1 cup vegetable broth or water
iii.   1 tablespoon olive oil
iv.   Salt and pepper to taste

Instructions:

For the Tagine:

i.   **Heat the Olive Oil:** In a large tagine or a heavy-bottomed pot, heat the olive oil over medium heat.

ii. **Sauté Aromatics:** Add the finely chopped onion and sauté until it becomes translucent, about 3-4 minutes. Stir in the minced garlic and ginger and cook for another minute until fragrant.

iii. **Spice it Up:** Add the ground cumin, ground coriander, ground paprika, ground cinnamon, and cayenne pepper to the pot. Stir well to coat the onion mixture with the spices. Cook for 1-2 minutes to toast the spices, stirring constantly.

iv. **Add Vegetables:** Add the diced carrots, potatoes, zucchini, and red bell pepper to the pot. Stir to combine them with the spiced onion mixture.

v. **Chickpeas and Tomatoes:** Add the chickpeas and diced tomatoes (with their juice) to the pot. Mix everything together.

vi. **Add Broth:** Pour in the vegetable broth, which will help create a flavorful sauce. Season with salt and pepper to taste.

vii. **Simmer:** Reduce the heat to low, cover the tagine or pot, and let it simmer for about 20-25 minutes, or until the vegetables are tender and the flavors meld together. Stir occasionally to prevent sticking.

viii. **Garnish and Serve:** Garnish the Moroccan Chickpea Tagine with fresh cilantro or parsley before serving.

For the Couscous (optional):

i. **Prepare Couscous:** While the tagine is simmering, you can prepare couscous as a side dish. In a separate pot, bring the vegetable broth (or water) to a boil. Stir in the couscous, cover with a lid, and remove from heat. Let it sit for 5 minutes, then fluff with a fork. Use salt, olive oil and pepper to season.

Benefits of Moroccan Chickpea Tagine:

i. **High in Fiber:** Chickpeas are a great source of dietary fiber, which aids in digestion and helps maintain a feeling of fullness.

ii. **Protein:** Chickpeas are a good plant-based protein source, making this dish suitable for vegetarians and vegans.

iii. **Rich in Vitamins and Minerals:** The vegetables and spices in the tagine provide essential vitamins and minerals, including vitamin C, vitamin A, and various B vitamins.

iv. **Antioxidants:** The spices used in Moroccan cuisine, such as cumin, coriander, and cinnamon, are rich in antioxidants that help protect your cells from oxidative stress.

v. **Heart-Healthy:** This dish is low in saturated fats and cholesterol, which can contribute to heart health.

vi. **Delicious Flavor:** Moroccan Chickpea Tagine is known for its complex and aromatic flavors, making it a satisfying and enjoyable meal.

Moroccan Chickpea Tagine is a nutritious and flavorful dish that can be served with couscous or bread. It's a wonderful way to enjoy the exotic flavors of North African cuisine and provides numerous health benefits due to its wholesome ingredients.

2. Thai Green Curry:

Take a trip to Thailand with a creamy and aromatic Thai Green Curry. This dish features an enticing blend of coconut milk, green curry paste, and a variety of vegetables and tofu. The result is a flavorful and spicy curry that's perfectly served over jasmine rice.

How to Prepare:

Ingredients:

For the Green Curry Paste (you can also use store-bought):

i. 2-3 green Thai chilies, seeds removed (adjust to taste for spiciness)
ii. 2-3 cloves garlic, minced
iii. 1 small shallot, minced
iv. 1 lemongrass stalk, minced (tender parts only)
v. 1-inch piece of galangal or ginger, minced
vi. Zest and juice of 1 lime
vii. 1 tablespoon coriander seeds, toasted and ground
viii. Toasted and ground cumin seeds- 1 teaspoon
ix. 1/2 teaspoon white pepper
x. 1/2 teaspoon shrimp paste (omit for a vegetarian/vegan version)
xi. A handful of fresh cilantro leaves and stems
xii. 2-3 kaffir lime leaves, minced (optional)
xiii. 1 tablespoon vegetable oil

For the Curry:

i. 1 can (13.5 ounces) coconut milk (full-fat for creaminess)
ii. 2 tablespoons green curry paste (adjust to taste)
iii. 1 tablespoon vegetable oil

iv. 1 pound (450g) protein of your choice (e.g., chicken, tofu, shrimp)

v. 1 bell pepper, thinly sliced

vi. 1 zucchini, sliced into half-moons

vii. 1 cup green beans, trimmed and cut into bite-sized pieces

viii. 1-2 tablespoons fish sauce or soy sauce (adjust to taste)

ix. 1-2 teaspoons palm sugar or brown sugar (adjust to taste)

x. Fresh basil or cilantro leaves for garnish (optional)

xi. Cooked jasmine rice for serving

Instructions:

For the Green Curry Paste:

i. In a mortar and pestle or a food processor, combine all the green curry paste ingredients. Pound or process until you have a smooth paste. If needed, add a little water to help with blending.

For the Curry:

i. Over medium-high heat, heat the vegetable oil in wok or a large skillet. Then add the green curry paste. Stir continuously as you fry for 1-2 minutes until fragrant.

ii.	Add the protein of your choice (e.g., chicken, tofu, shrimp) and cook until it's browned or cooked through. If using tofu, ensure it's well browned on all sides.

iii.	Add the coconut milk. Mix well and boil the mixture gentlyssssss.

iv.	Add the sliced bell pepper, zucchini, and green beans to the simmering curry. Cook for 5-7 minutes or until the vegetables are tender but still crisp.

v.	Season the curry with fish sauce (or soy sauce) and palm sugar (or brown sugar) to taste. Adjust the seasoning to balance the flavors, adding more if necessary.

vi.	Remove the curry from heat and let it sit for a few minutes to allow the flavors to meld together.

vii.	Serve the Thai Green Curry over cooked jasmine rice. Garnish with fresh basil or cilantro leaves if desired.

Benefits of Thai Green Curry:

i.	**Aromatic and Flavorful:** Thai Green Curry is known for its aromatic and complex flavors, thanks to ingredients like lemongrass, galangal, kaffir lime leaves, and green chilies.

ii.   **Rich in Coconut Milk:** Coconut milk provides healthy fats and a creamy texture, contributing to the dish's richness.

iii.   **Vegetable and Protein Variety:** The curry is typically loaded with vegetables and can be customized with your choice of protein, making it a balanced meal.

iv.   **Spices and Herbs:** Many of the herbs and spices used in Thai Green Curry, such as coriander, cumin, and ginger, have potential health benefits due to their antioxidant properties.

v.   **Versatile:** You can adjust the spiciness and ingredients to suit your taste and dietary preferences, making it suitable for various diets, including vegetarian and vegan.

Thai Green Curry is not only delicious but also a colorful and nutritious dish. It's a delightful way to explore the flavors of Thai cuisine and enjoy a variety of vegetables and proteins in one meal.

3. Italian Eggplant Parmesan:

Italy's beloved Eggplant Parmesan gets a vegan makeover in this recipe. Slices of eggplant are coated in breadcrumbs, baked until crispy, and then layered with marinara sauce and vegan mozzarella.

The result is a comforting and satisfying dish that captures the essence of Italian cuisine.

How to Prepare:

Ingredients:

For the Eggplant:

i. 2 large eggplants
ii. Salt
iii. 2 cups breadcrumbs (you can use Italian-style breadcrumbs for extra flavor)
iv. 1 cup all-purpose flour
v. 3 large eggs
vi. Vegetable oil for frying

For the Tomato Sauce:

i. 2 cups tomato sauce (homemade or store-bought)
ii. 2 cloves garlic, minced
iii. Oregano leaves (dried)- 1 teaspoon
iv. 1 teaspoon dried basil
v. Salt and pepper to taste

For Assembly:

i. Mozzarella cheese (shredded)- 2 cups
ii. 1/2 cup grated Parmesan cheese
iii. Fresh basil or parsley leaves for garnish (optional)

Instructions:

Preparing the Eggplant:

i. Slice the eggplants into 1/4-inch thick rounds. Place the slices in a colander, sprinkling each layer with salt and allow them to sit for 30 minutes. This will help to remove bitterness and excess moisture from the eggplants.

ii. After 30 minutes, rinse the eggplant slices under cold water and pat them dry with paper towels.

iii. Take three shallow bowls. In one, add flour and beat the eggs in the second one, then in the third shallow bowl, place the breadcrumbs..

iv. Dip each eggplant slice first in the flour, then in the beaten eggs, and finally in the breadcrumbs, pressing the breadcrumbs onto the eggplant to adhere.

v. Over a medium-high heat, heat up vegetable oil in a large skillet and fry the eggplant (breaded) slices until they are golden brown on both sides. Then remove excess oil by placing them on paper towels.

Making the Tomato Sauce:

i. In a saucepan, heat a bit of olive oil over medium heat. Add the minced garlic and sauté until fragrant, about 1 minute.

ii. Add the tomato sauce, dried oregano, dried basil, salt, and pepper. Simmer for about 15-20 minutes, stirring occasionally, until the sauce thickens and the flavors meld together.

Assembling and Baking:

i. Preheat your oven to 375°F (190°C).

ii. In a baking dish, spread a thin layer of tomato sauce on the bottom.

iii. Layer the fried eggplant slices on top of the sauce.

iv. Sprinkle shredded mozzarella cheese and grated Parmesan cheese over the eggplant slices.

v. Repeat the layers until you've used all your ingredients, finishing with a layer of cheese on top.

vi. Bake in the preheated oven for 25-30 minutes or until the cheese is bubbly and golden brown.

vii. Take out the cheese from the oven. Let it cool for some minutes before serving.

Benefits of Italian Eggplant Parmesan:

i. **Vegetable-Rich:** Eggplant is the star of this dish, and it's a low-calorie vegetable that's a good source of fiber and various vitamins and minerals.

ii. **Dietary Fiber:** The eggplant and tomato sauce provide dietary fiber, which supports healthy digestion.

iii. **Protein:** The cheese used in Eggplant Parmesan provides a source of protein, which is important for muscle and tissue repair.

iv. **Lycopene:** Tomatoes used in the sauce contain lycopene, a powerful antioxidant that may help protect against certain diseases.

v. **Calcium:** Parmesan cheese is a source of calcium, which is essential for strong bones and teeth.

vi. **Comfort Food:** Italian Eggplant Parmesan is a comforting and satisfying dish that's perfect for family gatherings or when you're in the mood for classic Italian flavors.

Italian Eggplant Parmesan is a delicious and hearty dish that showcases the flavors of Italy. It's a great way to enjoy eggplant and indulge in the cheesy goodness of traditional Italian cuisine. Serve it with a side of pasta or a simple green salad for a complete meal.

4. Japanese Veggie Sushi:

Bring the art of sushi-making into your kitchen with Japanese Veggie Sushi. Sushi rice is paired with fresh vegetables, avocado, and tofu, then rolled in nori seaweed sheets. Serve with soy sauce, wasabi, and pickled ginger for an authentic Japanese experience.

How to Prepare:

Ingredients:

For the Sushi Rice:

    i.   1 cup sushi rice (short-grain Japanese rice)
    ii.   2 cups water
    iii.   1/4 cup rice vinegar
    iv.   2 tablespoons sugar
    v.   1/2 teaspoon salt

For the Sushi Filling (options; choose your favorites):

    i.   Cucumber, thinly sliced into strips
    ii.   Avocado, thinly sliced
    iii.   Carrots, peeled and thinly julienned
    iv.   Bell peppers, thinly sliced
    v.   Radishes, thinly sliced

vi.   Scallions (green onions), thinly sliced lengthwise

vii.   Firm tofu, sliced and marinated in soy sauce

viii.   Pickled ginger (gari)

ix.   Wasabi paste

x.   Soy sauce or tamari for dipping

For Assembly:

i.   Nori sheets (seaweed wrappers)

ii.   Bamboo sushi rolling mat (makisu)

iii.   Plastic wrap

Instructions:

For the Sushi Rice:

i.   Rinse the sushi rice under cold water until the water runs clear.

ii.   In a medium saucepan, combine the rinsed rice and 2 cups of water. Bring to a boil, then reduce the heat to low, cover, and simmer for about 15-20 minutes, or until the rice is cooked and the water is absorbed.

iii.   While the rice is cooking, in a small saucepan, heat the rice vinegar, sugar, and salt over low heat, stirring until the sugar and salt are completely dissolved. Remove from heat and let it cool.

iv. When the rice is done, transfer it to a large mixing bowl. Gradually add the vinegar mixture to the rice, gently folding it in to combine. Allow the rice to cool to room temperature.

For Assembly:

i. Place a bamboo sushi rolling mat (makisu) on a clean, flat surface. Lay a sheet of plastic wrap over the mat to prevent sticking.

ii. Lay a sheet of nori, shiny side down, on the plastic wrap.

iii. Wet your fingers with water to prevent the rice from sticking. Take a handful of sushi rice and evenly spread it over the nori, leaving a small border along the top edge.

iv. Arrange your choice of vegetables or tofu in the center of the rice.

v. Carefully lift the bamboo mat and the edge of the nori closest to you, and start rolling the nori and rice over the filling. Use gentle pressure to shape the roll.

vi. Continue rolling until you reach the uncovered edge of the nori. Wet the exposed edge with a little water and press to seal the sushi roll.

vii. Using a sharp knife dipped in water, slice the sushi roll into bite-sized pieces.

viii. Repeat the process with the remaining nori sheets and fillings.

Benefits of Japanese Veggie Sushi:

i. **Low in Calories:** Japanese Veggie Sushi is generally low in calories, making it a healthy option for those looking to manage their calorie intake.

ii. **Rich in Vegetables:** This dish is loaded with fresh vegetables, providing essential vitamins, minerals, and dietary fiber.

iii. **Plant-Based:** Veggie sushi is entirely plant-based, making it suitable for vegetarians and vegans.

iv. **Heart-Healthy:** The vegetables and rice are naturally low in fat, and the addition of avocado provides healthy fats, which can support heart health.

v. **Gluten-Free Option:** If you use gluten-free soy sauce (tamari) and ensure the nori and other ingredients are gluten-free, veggie sushi can be a suitable option for those with gluten sensitivities.

vi. **Customizable:** You can customize your veggie sushi with your favorite vegetables and seasonings, making it a versatile and satisfying meal.

Japanese Veggie Sushi is not only delicious but also a visually appealing and healthy option for those seeking a plant-based meal or a lighter sushi option. It's a fun and creative dish to prepare at home and can be enjoyed as a snack, appetizer, or main course. Serve it with soy sauce, pickled ginger, and wasabi for the complete sushi experience.

5. Mexican Enchiladas:

Spice things up with Mexican Enchiladas, featuring corn tortillas filled with a savory mixture of black beans, sautéed vegetables, and smothered in spicy enchilada sauce. Top with vegan cheese and bake until bubbly for a satisfying Mexican feast.

How to Prepare:

Ingredients:

For the Enchiladas:

i.   8-10 corn tortillas (you can also use flour tortillas)

ii. 2 cups cooked and shredded chicken (optional for meat lovers)

iii. 1 cup cooked and mashed black beans (vegetarian option)

iv. 1 cup shredded cheese (cheddar, Monterey Jack, or your choice)

v.   1/2 cup diced onions

vi. 1/2 cup chopped fresh cilantro

vii.   Vegetable oil for frying tortillas (if desired)

viii.   Sour cream and additional cilantro for garnish (optional)

For the Enchilada Sauce:

i.   2 cups tomato sauce or canned crushed tomatoes

ii.   2 cloves garlic, minced

iii.   1 teaspoon ground cumin

iv.   1 teaspoon chili powder

v.   1/2 teaspoon dried oregano

vi.   Salt and pepper to taste

vii.   1-2 tablespoons vegetable oil for sautéing

Instructions:

For the Enchilada Sauce:

i.   Over medium heat, heat vegetable oil in a saucepan. Then add minced garlic and fry while stirring continuously for about 30 seconds until fragrant.

ii.   Add the tomato sauce or crushed tomatoes, ground cumin, chili powder, dried oregano, salt, and pepper. Stir well to combine.

iii.   Simmer the sauce for about 10-15 minutes, stirring occasionally. Adjust the seasoning to taste.

iv. Remove the sauce from heat and set it aside.

For the Enchiladas:

i. Preheat your oven to 350°F (175°C).

ii. If using corn tortillas, fry each one lightly in a vegetable oil for a few seconds on each side you can soften them and then drain it of oil on paper towels. If using flour tortillas, you can skip this step.

iii. In a mixing bowl, combine the shredded chicken (if using), mashed black beans, diced onions, and chopped cilantro. Mix well.

iv. Warm the tortillas in the microwave or on a skillet to make them pliable.

v. Take a tortilla, place a spoonful of the filling mixture down the center, and roll it up tightly. Place it seam-side down in a baking dish. Repeat with the remaining tortillas and filling.

vi. Pour the enchilada sauce over the rolled tortillas, making sure they are evenly coated.

vii. Sprinkle the shredded cheese over the top of the enchiladas.

viii. Bake in the preheated oven for about 20-25 minutes, or until the cheese is melted and the enchiladas are heated through.

ix. Garnish the enchiladas with sour cream and additional chopped cilantro if desired.

Benefits of Mexican Enchiladas:

i. **Protein:** Enchiladas can be a good source of protein, whether you use chicken, beans, or a combination of both as your filling.

ii. **Fiber-Rich:** Black beans, a common ingredient in Mexican cuisine, are rich in dietary fiber, which aids in digestion and helps maintain a feeling of fullness.

iii. **Vitamins and Minerals:** Ingredients like onions, cilantro, and tomatoes provide essential vitamins and minerals, including vitamin C, vitamin K, and potassium.

iv. **Spices and Flavor:** Mexican cuisine incorporates a variety of spices and herbs, such as cumin and chili powder, which can have potential health benefits and add flavor to the dish.

v. **Customizable:** You can customize your enchiladas with your favorite fillings, making them versatile and suitable for various dietary preferences.

vi. **Comfort Food:** Mexican Enchiladas are a comforting and satisfying dish, perfect for family meals or when you're craving flavorful, hearty food.

Mexican Enchiladas are a delicious and versatile dish that can be customized to suit your taste. Whether you prefer them with meat, beans, or vegetables, they're a crowd-pleaser and a great way to enjoy the flavors of Mexican cuisine. Enjoy them as a main course or serve them as part of a larger Mexican feast.

6. Mediterranean Chickpea and Couscous Bowl:

Mediterranean Chickpea and Couscous Bowl is a vibrant and flavorful dish that brings together a variety of ingredients commonly found in Mediterranean cuisine. It's a balanced and wholesome meal that combines grains, legumes, vegetables, and Mediterranean-inspired flavors. Here's a description of what you might find in a Mediterranean Chickpea and Couscous Bowl

How to Prepare:

Ingredients:

For the Couscous:

    i.   1 cup whole wheat couscous
    ii.   1 1/4 cups vegetable broth
    iii.   Olive oil- a tablespoon
    iv.   1/2 teaspoon ground cumin
    v.   Salt and pepper to taste

For the Chickpea Mixture:

    i.   2 (15 oz) cans chickpeas, drained and rinsed

    ii.   2 tablespoons olive oil

    iii.   2 minced cloves of garlic

    iv.   1 teaspoon ground cumin

    v.   1/2 teaspoon smoked paprika

    vi.   Salt and pepper to taste

For Toppings:

    i.   Cucumber, diced

    ii.   Cherry tomatoes, halved

    iii.   Kalamata olives, pitted and sliced

    iv.   Red onion, finely chopped

    v.   Fresh parsley, chopped

    vi.   Hummus (store-bought or homemade)

    vii.   Lemon wedges

Instructions:

For the Couscous:

    i.   In a saucepan, bring the vegetable broth, olive oil, ground cumin, salt, and pepper to a boil.

    ii.   Stir in the couscous, cover, and remove from heat. Let it sit for 5 minutes, then fluff with a fork.

For the Chickpea Mixture:

i.   In a skillet, heat the olive oil over medium heat.

ii.   Add the minced garlic and fry while stirring until it's fragrant.

iii.   Stir in the chickpeas, ground cumin, smoked paprika, salt, and pepper. Cook for 5-7 minutes until heated through.

To Assemble:

i.   Divide the cooked couscous among serving bowls.

ii.   Top with the chickpea mixture.

iii.   Garnish with diced cucumber, cherry tomatoes, Kalamata olives, red onion, and fresh parsley.

iv.   Serve with hummus and lemon wedges on the side.

Benefits:

i.   **Plant-Based Protein:** Chickpeas provide a good source of plant-based protein, aiding in muscle repair and overall health.

ii.   **Whole Grains:** Whole wheat couscous offers complex carbohydrates and dietary fiber, promoting sustained energy.

iii.   Mediterranean Flavors: Ingredients like olives and olive oil contribute healthy fats and a Mediterranean-inspired taste.

7.

Conclusion:

Chapter 9 guided you through a global culinary adventure that celebrates the diverse and flavorful world of international vegan cuisine. These recipes capture the essence of each region's culinary traditions, allowing you to savor the exotic flavors and aromas from around the world, all while aligning with your plant-based lifestyle. So, gather your ingredients and embrace the international flavors that will transport your taste buds to far-off places.

Veggie Delights

Chapter 10:

Hearty Vegan Bowls.

This last chapter brings you the concept of Hearty Vegan Bowls, a modern culinary trend that combines balanced nutrition with an explosion of flavors and textures. These bowls are not just visually appealing but also offer a wholesome and satisfying way to enjoy a complete meal in a single dish. From Buddha bowls to grain bowls and protein-packed power bowls, this chapter introduces you to a world of customizable creations that cater to your taste and dietary preferences.

1. **Buddha Bowls:** Buddha bowls are a celebration of balance and harmony. These colorful and nutrient-rich bowls typically consist of a base (such as brown rice, quinoa, or couscous), a variety of cooked and raw vegetables, plant-based protein (like tofu or chickpeas), and a flavorful sauce or dressing. The result is a visually stunning and nourishing bowl that offers a medley of flavors and textures in every bite.

How to Prepare:

Ingredients:

The beauty of Buddha Bowls is that they are highly customizable, and you can use a wide range of ingredients based on your preferences and what's available. Here are some typical components:

i. **Grains (Base):** Cooked quinoa, brown rice, farro, couscous, or any other whole grain of your choice.

ii. **Proteins:** Baked or grilled chicken, tofu, tempeh, chickpeas, black beans, lentils, or any other protein source you prefer.

iii. **Vegetables (Roasted, Raw, or Pickled):** Roasted sweet potatoes, broccoli, cauliflower, carrots, or any vegetables you like.
Fresh greens like spinach, kale, arugula, or mixed salad greens.
Sliced cucumber, cherry tomatoes, bell peppers, radishes, or any fresh veggies you enjoy.
Pickled vegetables like red onions, beets, or cabbage for added flavor.

iv. **Healthy Fats:**
Avocado slices, diced avocado, or guacamole.
Nuts and seeds such as almonds, pumpkin seeds, or sesame seeds.

v. **Dressings and Sauces:**
Tahini sauce, homemade vinaigrette, yogurt-based dressings, or your favorite sauce to drizzle over the bowl.

vi. **Garnishes:**
Fresh herbs like cilantro, parsley, or basil. Sliced scallions, sesame seeds, or microgreens.

Instructions:

i. **Prepare the Base:** Start by cooking your chosen grain according to the package instructions. Fluff the cooked grain with a fork and divide it into serving bowls, creating a base for your Buddha Bowl.

ii. **Proteins:** Cook your protein source (e.g., grilled chicken, tofu, chickpeas) as desired. Season it with your favorite herbs and spices for added flavor.

iii. **Vegetables:** Prepare your vegetables. Roast them in the oven with a drizzle of olive oil, salt, and pepper, or keep them raw and fresh. You can also include pickled vegetables for a tangy element.

iv. **Healthy Fats:** Slice or dice avocado, or prepare your choice of nuts and seeds. These provide healthy fats and a satisfying crunch.

v. **Dressings and Sauces:** Prepare a dressing or sauce of your choice. Tahini-based dressings, balsamic vinaigrettes, and yogurt-based sauces are popular options.

Adjust the dressing to your desired consistency and taste.

Assemble the Bowl:

Start by arranging the grains at the base of each bowl. Next, add your chosen proteins, followed by the vegetables and healthy fats. Drizzle the dressing or sauce over the top.

i. **Garnish:** Sprinkle fresh herbs, scallions, and seeds on top for added flavor and texture.

ii. **Serve:** Buddha Bowls are typically served immediately, either warm or at room temperature.

Benefits of Buddha Bowls:

i. **Nutrient-Dense:** Buddha Bowls are packed with a variety of colorful, fresh, and whole foods, providing a wide range of essential nutrients, vitamins, and minerals.

ii. **Balanced Meal:** These bowls naturally offer a balance of macronutrients, including carbohydrates, proteins, and healthy fats, promoting sustained energy levels and satiety.

iii. **High in Fiber:** Whole grains and vegetables provide dietary fiber, supporting digestive health and helping you feel full and satisfied.

iv. **Customizable:** You can personalize Buddha Bowls to suit your dietary preferences, making them suitable for vegetarians, vegans, gluten-free diets, and more.

v. **Versatile:** Buddha Bowls are versatile and can be adapted to use seasonal ingredients or to help reduce food waste by using leftovers.

vi. **Visual Appeal:** The colorful and beautifully arranged ingredients in a Buddha Bowl make it a visually appealing and enjoyable meal.

vii. **Sustainability:** By using locally sourced, seasonal ingredients, Buddha Bowls can be a sustainable meal choice that reduces the environmental footprint.

Buddha Bowls offer a delightful way to nourish your body with a wide array of flavors, textures, and nutrients. They encourage creativity in the kitchen and are an excellent option for busy individuals looking for a convenient, balanced, and healthful meal.

2. **Grain Bowls:**

Grain bowls focus on the wholesome goodness of whole grains. Start with your choice of grains, such as farro, bulgur, or barley, and layer them with a selection of roasted or sautéed vegetables, legumes, and herbs. These bowls are known for their heartiness and are often topped with a drizzle of tahini, balsamic glaze, or a citrus vinaigrette for added depth of flavor.

How to Prepare:

Ingredients:

i. **Base Grain:**
Choose your preferred whole grain as the base. Options include brown rice, quinoa, farro, bulgur, barley, or couscous.

ii. **Vegetables:**
A mix of fresh, roasted, steamed, or sautéed vegetables adds color and nutrients. Common choices include spinach, kale, broccoli, carrots, bell peppers, cherry tomatoes, cucumbers, and avocados.

iii. **Proteins:**
Select a protein source to add substance to your bowl. Options include:
Grilled or roasted chicken, turkey, or tofu
Beans (e.g., black beans, chickpeas, kidney beans)

Lentils
Salmon, tuna, or other fish
Shrimp
Eggs (boiled, fried, or poached)

iv. **Healthy Fats:**
Include sources of healthy fats for flavor and satiety. Avocado slices, nuts like almonds and walnuts, seeds like sesame seeds and pumpkin seeds. A drizzle of olive oil are great choices.

v. **Dressing or Sauce:**
A flavorful dressing or sauce ties the bowl together. Options include vinaigrettes, tahini-based dressings, soy-based sauces, yogurt-based sauces, or your favorite homemade sauce.

vi. **Toppings:**
Add extra texture and flavor with toppings like fresh herbs (e.g., cilantro, basil, parsley), crumbled cheese (e.g., feta, goat cheese), dried fruits (e.g., cranberries, raisins), or grated Parmesan.

Instructions:

i. **Prepare the Base Grain:** Cook the chosen grain according to the package instructions. Typically, it involves boiling, simmering, or steaming until the grains are tender. Fluff the grains with a fork when done.

ii. **Cook the Protein:** Cook your chosen protein source like fish, beans, chicken, tofu, or lentils to your preferred taste. Seasoning and flavoring are as you desire.

iii. **Prepare the Vegetables:** Wash, chop, and prepare the vegetables. You can roast or sauté some for added flavor and texture, while others can be left raw for crunch and freshness.

iv. **Make the Dressing or Sauce:** Prepare your dressing or sauce by whisking together the ingredients in a bowl. Adjust the flavors to your liking.

v. **Assemble the Bowl:** Start with a generous portion of cooked grain as the base of your bowl.

vi. Arrange your cooked protein, vegetables, and healthy fats (e.g., avocado, nuts, seeds) around the grain.

vii. Drizzle your chosen dressing or sauce over the top.s

viii. **Add Toppings**: Sprinkle your choice of toppings, such as fresh herbs, cheese, dried fruits, or grated Parmesan, over the bowl for extra flavor and texture.

ix. **Serve:** Enjoy your grain bowl immediately while it's fresh and flavorful.

Benefits of Grain Bowls:

i. **Nutrient Density:** Grain bowls are packed with a variety of nutrient-rich ingredients, providing essential vitamins, minerals, and antioxidants.

ii. **Balanced Nutrition:** They offer a balanced combination of carbohydrates (from grains), protein (from various sources), healthy fats (from avocado, nuts, and seeds), and fiber (from vegetables and grains).

iii. **Customizable:** You can tailor grain bowls to meet your dietary preferences, including vegetarian, vegan, gluten-free, and low-carb options.

iv. **Satiety:** The balanced mix of nutrients and fiber helps keep you full and satisfied, making grain bowls a great choice for a filling meal.

v. **Versatility:** Grain bowls are incredibly versatile, allowing you to use seasonal ingredients, leftovers, or whatever you have on hand to create a satisfying meal.

vi. **Convenience:** They are easy to prepare, making them suitable for quick, wholesome weeknight dinners or packed lunches.

Grain bowls are not only nutritious and convenient but also a delightful way to enjoy a wide variety of flavors and textures in one meal. Experiment with different ingredients and flavor combinations to create your favorite grain bowl recipes.

3. **Protein-Packed Power Bowls:**

For those looking to fuel an active lifestyle or build muscle on a plant-based diet, Protein-Packed Power Bowls are the way to go. These bowls feature high-protein components like quinoa, tempeh, edamame, or lentils paired with a variety of vegetables and a creamy hummus or avocado dressing. They provide an energy boost and are perfect for post-workout refueling.

How to Prepare:

Ingredients:

i. **Protein Source:**
   Choose a protein-rich component as the focal point of your bowl. Options include:
   - Grilled or roasted chicken, turkey, or tofu
   - Lean beef, pork, or fish (salmon, tuna, etc.)
   - Plant-based proteins like tempeh, seitan, or edamame
   - Legumes (e.g., beans, lentils, chickpeas)

ii. **Whole Grains:** Select a whole grain as the base of your bowl. Whole grains

provide complex carbohydrates and fiber. Options include:
Brown rice, Quinoa, Farro, Bulgur, Barley, Whole wheat couscous

iii. **Vegetables:** Include a variety of vegetables for color, flavor, and essential nutrients. Common choices are:
- Leafy greens (e.g., spinach, kale, arugula), Bell peppers, Cherry tomatoes, Cucumbers, steamed broccoli, Avocado, Sliced carrots

iv. **Healthy Fats:** Incorporate sources of healthy fats for satiety and flavor. Options include:
- Avocado slices or guacamole, Nuts (e.g., almonds, walnuts), Seeds (e.g., chia seeds, pumpkin seeds)

v. **Dressing or Sauce:** Prepare a flavorful dressing or sauce to tie all the ingredients together. Options include vinaigrettes, tahini-based dressings, yogurt-based sauces, or your favorite homemade sauce.

vi. **Toppings:** Add toppings for extra texture and flavor, such as crumbled cheese (e.g., feta, goat cheese), fresh herbs (e.g., cilantro, basil), dried fruits (e.g., cranberries, raisins), or grated Parmesan.

Instructions:

Prepare the Protein:

Veggie Delights

i. Cook your chosen protein source (e.g., chicken, tofu, beans, lentils, fish) according to your preference. Season and flavor as desired.

ii. Cook the Whole Grains:

iii. Cook the selected whole grain according to the package instructions. Typically, it involves boiling, simmering, or steaming until the grains are tender. Fluff the grains with a fork when done.

Prepare the Vegetables:

i. Wash, chop, and prepare the vegetables. You can roast or sauté some for added flavor and texture, while others can be left raw for crunch and freshness.

ii. Make the Dressing or Sauce:

Prepare your dressing or sauce by whisking together the ingredients in a bowl. You have to adjust the flavors to your taste.

Assemble the Bowl:

i. Start with a generous portion of cooked whole grains as the base of your bowl.

ii. Arrange your cooked protein, vegetables, and healthy fats (e.g., avocado, nuts, seeds) around the grain.

iii. Drizzle your chosen dressing or sauce over the top.

iv. **Add Toppings:** Sprinkle your choice of toppings, such as fresh herbs, cheese, dried fruits, or grated Parmesan, over the bowl for extra flavor and texture.

v. **Serve:** Enjoy your Protein-Packed Power Bowl immediately while it's fresh and flavorful.

Benefits of Protein-Packed Power Bowls:

i. **High Protein Content:** These bowls are designed to provide a substantial amount of protein, which is essential for muscle maintenance and overall body function.

ii. **Balanced Nutrition:** They offer a balanced combination of carbohydrates (from whole grains), protein (from various sources), healthy fats (from avocado, nuts, and seeds), and fiber (from vegetables and grains).

iii. **Satiety:** The balanced mix of nutrients, including protein and fiber, helps keep you full and satisfied, making Protein-Packed Power Bowls an ideal choice for a filling meal.

iv. **Customizable:** You can tailor these bowls to meet your dietary preferences, including vegetarian, vegan, gluten-free, and low-carb options.

v. **Versatility:** Protein-Packed Power Bowls are incredibly versatile, allowing you to use seasonal ingredients, leftovers, or whatever you have on hand to create a satisfying meal.

vi. **Convenience:** They are easy to prepare, making them suitable for quick, wholesome weeknight dinners or packed lunches.

vii. **Protein-Packed**: Power Bowls are a delicious and nutritious way to provide your body with the protein and essential nutrients it needs. Experiment with different ingredients and flavor combinations to create your favorite power bowl recipes.

4. **Sweet and Savory Breakfast Bowls:**

Breakfast takes center stage with Sweet and Savory Breakfast Bowls. These morning delights feature a base of oats, quinoa, or chia pudding topped with a creative combination of fruits, nuts, seeds, and sweet or savory toppings. Whether you're in the mood for a hearty breakfast or a refreshing acai bowl, these creations ensure your day starts on the right note.

How to Prepare:

Veggie Delights

Ingredients:

i. 1/2 cup of cooked quinoa, oats, or another grain of your choice (such as rice or farro)

ii. 1/4 cup of Greek yogurt or dairy-free alternative (for creaminess)

iii. 1/4 cup of milk (dairy or non-dairy)

iv. 1/4 teaspoon of vanilla extract (for sweet bowls)

v. 1 teaspoon of honey or maple syrup (for sweet bowls)

vi. A pinch of salt

vii. A pinch of ground cinnamon (optional)

viii. Sweet Toppings (choose your favorites):

ix. Sliced bananas

x. Berries (strawberries, blueberries, raspberries)

xi. Sliced peaches or nectarines

xii. Chopped nuts (almonds, walnuts, or pecans)

xiii. Dried fruits (raisins, cranberries)

xiv. Chia seeds or flax seeds

xv. A drizzle of honey or maple syrup

xvi. Nut butter (peanut, almond, or cashew)

xvii. Savory Toppings (choose your favorites):

xviii. Sautéed spinach or kale

xix. Sliced avocado

xx. Sautéed mushrooms

xxi. Cherry tomatoes, halved

xxii. Soft-boiled or fried eggs

xxiii. Sliced scallions or chives

xxiv. Grated cheese (cheddar, feta, or parmesan)

xxv. Crispy bacon or cooked sausage (optional)

xxvi. Hot sauce or salsa (for some heat)

Instructions

Cook the Grains: Prepare your chosen grain (quinoa, oats, rice, etc.) according to package instructions and set aside.

i. **Sweet or Savory Base:** In a mixing bowl, combine the cooked grains with the milk, Greek yogurt (for creaminess), a pinch of salt, and vanilla extract and honey (for sweet bowls). For savory bowls, omit the sweet ingredients.

ii. **Mix Well:** Stir the mixture thoroughly until it's well combined. You can adjust the consistency by adding more milk if needed.

iii. **Toppings:** For sweet bowls, layer your chosen sweet toppings over the creamy base. For savory bowls, prepare and add your savory toppings.

iv. **Garnish:** Add any additional garnishes, such as a drizzle of honey, a sprinkle of cinnamon, or a dollop of nut butter (for sweet bowls) or herbs (for savory bowls).

v. **Enjoy:** Dive in and enjoy your delicious sweet or savory breakfast bowl!

Benefits of Sweet and Savory Breakfast Bowls:

i. **Balanced Nutrition:** Sweet and savory breakfast bowls offer a balanced combination of carbohydrates, protein, and healthy fats, helping to keep you full and energized throughout the morning.

ii. **Versatility:** You can customize these bowls to suit your dietary preferences and nutritional needs. Whether you're vegetarian, vegan, or omnivorous, there's a breakfast bowl variation for you.

iii. **Nutrient-Rich:** Depending on your toppings, these bowls can be rich in vitamins, minerals, and antioxidants. Berries provide vitamins and fiber, while avocado offers healthy fats and potassium.

iv. **Satiety:** The combination of grains, yogurt, and toppings provides a satisfying and filling breakfast that can help reduce mid-morning snacking.

v. **Digestive Health:** Adding fiber-rich ingredients like chia seeds and fruits to your breakfast can support digestive health and regularity.

vi. **Quick and Easy:** Breakfast bowls are quick to prepare and allow for creativity in the kitchen. You can mix and match ingredients to suit your taste and time constraints.

vii. **Flavor Variety:** Sweet and savory bowls offer a wide range of flavors, ensuring you never get bored with your morning meal.

Remember to tailor your breakfast bowl to your personal preferences and dietary needs. Whether you're craving a sweet treat or a savory delight, these bowls offer a satisfying and nutritious way to kick start your day.

Conclusion:

This chapter made you to embrace the world of Hearty Vegan Bowls, where nutrition and flavor unite in a single, delightful dish. These recipes provide a canvas for your culinary creativity, allowing you to customize your bowls according to your taste preferences and dietary requirements. Whether you're seeking a wholesome lunch, a post-workout meal, or a vibrant breakfast, these bowls offer a versatile and satisfying way to enjoy plant-based eating. So, gather your ingredients, mix and match to your heart's content, and create Hearty

Veggie Delights

Vegan Bowls that cater to both your palate and your well-being.

Veggie Delights

Conclusion

Thus far, it can be confidently said that this cookbook, "Veggie Delights: A Collection of Mouthwatering Vegan Recipes" succeeded in pushing the conventional boundaries of vegan cuisine. It has also succeeded in proving that plant-based meals can be as satisfying, if not more, than regular meals. I believe that the presentation of the diverse and appealing recipes in this cookbook was engaging and worthwhile. The intention is to encourage a shift towards more compassionate, healthier, and more environmentally friendly eating.

With "Veggie Delights", the future of the culinary world appears to be not only green but also extremely delicious. Wishing you happy and delicious cooking!

www.ingramcontent.com/pod-product-compliance
Lightning Source LLC
Chambersburg PA
CBHW050808260726
48660CB00004B/1319